Chicken Soup

& · OTHER · FOLK · REMEDIES ·

Other books by Joan Wilen and Lydia Wilen:
More Chicken Soup & Other Folk Remedies (Ballantine Books)
Folk Remedies That Work (HarperCollins)
Garlic—Nature's Super Healer (Prentice Hall)
Shoes in the Freezer, Beer in the Flower Bed
(Simon & Schuster)
The Perfect Name for the Perfect Baby (Fawcett Columbine)

Chicken Soup

& · OTHER · FOLK · REMEDIES ·

revised edition

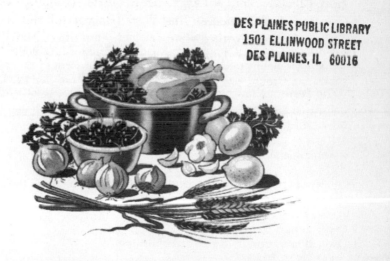

JOAN WILEN AND LYDIA WILEN

Ballantine Books · New York

The information contained in this book is based upon the research and experiences of the authors and the many contributors who shared their experiences and expertise. It is not intended as a substitute for consulting with your health-care provider.

The publisher and authors are not responsible for any consequences resulting from the use of any of the suggestions or preparations discussed in this book. All matters pertaining to your physical health should be supervised by your health-care professional.

Seeking more than one or two opinions is not a sign of insecurity, but a sign of wisdom.

A Ballantine Book
The Ballantine Publishing Group

Copyright © 1984, 2000 by Joan Wilen and Lydia Wilen
Illustrations copyright © 1984 by Elizabeth Koda-Callan

www.randomhouse.com

Library of Congress Catalog Card Number is available from the publisher upon request.

Cover design by Min Choi
Cover illustration by Gamboa Publishing

Manufactured in the United States of America

Revised Edition: September 2000

10 9 8 7 6 5 4 3 2 1

Chicken Soup & Other Folk Remedies
is dedicated to the loving memory of our parents,
Lillian and Jack Wilen—
Mom, who made the best chicken soup
in the whole wide world!
and Dad, who insisted we wear
camphor squares around our necks!

Contents

REMEDIES

Acknowledgments

A big thank-you to all the people who offered us their loving support, good wishes, and remedies:

Harry Wilen, Betty and Morris Wilen, Mina and Hy Wilen, Ann and Linda Iris Wilen, Roger Yager, Laura Yager, Dr. Ann Wigmore, Mary Pat Werner, Robert Weinstein, Gene, Anne and Theresa Vilfordi, Chris Verveniotis, Gwen Verdon, Judy Twersky, Vita Thalrose, Thelma Taylor, Margaret Sunshine, David Stanford, Esther Spitzer, Bill Smiddy, Rudy Shur, Gloria and Sidney R. Seltzer, Michael Sedgwick, Ellen and Fred Schreiber, Johnny Saltos, Dr. Norman and Susan Ruttner, Hilda and Moses Rosner, Patricia Riley, Rev. Thomas J. Ralph, Chipp Prosnit, Richard Perozzi, Eileen Pinsker, Ann and Joe Paull, Robert Pardi, Diana Okula, Eileen Nock, George Nider, Martha Neag, Dr. Marie Neag, John Nathan, Judy Montague, Blanche Miller, Bill McHugh, Frank McHale, Nick Malekos, Sheila Lukins, Countess Bianca Lovatelli, Gary Louisa, Mia Lottringer, Randie Levine, Paul David Levine, Mimi Levine, Ruth Lesser, Wendy and Jonathon Lazear, Ruth Landa, Helen and Larry Koster, Minnie Koskowitz, Jane and Bill Katz, Arleen and Anthony Kane, Lilly and Lester Kahn, Dr. Ronald N. Jones, Gene Stanley Jones, Eric Stephen Jacobs, Sylvia Holzberg, Dr. Ronald Hoffman, Suki, Elaine, Tina and Hy Hill, Angela Harris, Werner Haas, Libby Gurian, Veerani Gunavardhana, Mary Lynn and Howard Gottfried, Frances Goldstein, Barry Goldsmith, Walter Gidaly, Ronald E. Franzmeier, Vic Fiore, Thelma Felcher, Ray and Charles Farin, Rev. Lee Domez, B.J. DeSimone, Naomi Davis, James Daniels, Dorothy Conway, Becky and Brian Clement, James Chotas, Fung Wing Chin, Diana Chesmel, Morrie Buttnick, Miles P. Burton, Patricia Burke, Helen Burgess, Mildred Borofsky, Hank Blumfarb, Bill Mason Bivens, France Anthony Benko, Marlene Hope Ascherman, Sheila Anderson and Mollie Adler.

Special thanks to Mary Ellen Pinkham, to whom we will always be grateful for giving us our first chance in publishing.

For giving us a second chance, our gratitude goes to editor Leona Nevler.

Thanks also to Joelle Delbourgo, Michelle Russell, and Beth Heinsohn for nurturing this project.

For this new millennium version, extra special thanks to our wonderful editor, Elizabeth Zack. And to Rachel Tarlow-Gul for her support.

To a medical doctor who knows the value of nutritional/preventive medicine, Ray C. Wunderlich, Jr., M.D., B.A., M.A., Ph.D. candidate, P.A., we add "G.G." because he is one of the "Good Guys." We are very grateful to Dr. Wunderlich for his expert input.

Authors' Note
To Our Readers

"Doctor, I have a sore throat."

2000 B.C.: "Here, eat this root."

1000 B.C.: "That root is heathen. Say this prayer."

A.D. 1850 "That prayer is superstition. Drink this potion."

A.D. 1940: "That potion is snake oil. Swallow this pill."

A.D. 1980: "That pill is artificial and ineffective. Take this antibiotic."

A.D. 2000: "That antibiotic is artificial, causes bad side effects, and you've built an immunity to it. Take this root!"

And so we've gone back to our roots. Being city dwellers, we get our roots at herb shops and health food stores. Actually, that's not all that we get there. We take advantage of modern-day technology, and buy vitamins and other supplements that are commercially manufactured. You'll notice that along with the classic folk remedies in this book, we've added new remedies that may have *you* going to a health food store.

In this new millennium, we've come to realize that we have lots of choices when it comes to health care. It shouldn't be a matter of *alternative medicine* vs. *allopathic medicine*. Dr. Andrew Weil introduced us to the phrase *integrative medicine*, which combines traditional practices with alternative health treatments. Learn your options and, with the supervision of your health professional, take the best of both.

Joan and Lydia

Introduction

When we first signed the contract for the original edition of *Chicken Soup & Other Folk Remedies*, we went to all our relatives, asking for their home remedies. We heard wonderful "old-country" stories about remarkable cures, but times and places have changed dramatically. Going to the outskirts of Lomza Gubernia in Russia-Poland to pick *bopka blettles* is no longer practical. And we knew we wanted this book to not only be SAFE and EFFECTIVE, but PRACTICAL, too.

Yes, PRACTICAL! Every herb, fruit, vegetable, vitamin, mineral and liquid—in fact, all the ingredients mentioned in the book—can be bought at your local health food store, supermarket, or greengrocer—that is, if they aren't already in your home.

Our directions are easy to follow and, for the most part, specific. If exact amounts are not indicated, it means we could not find them, but we thought the remedy was important enough to include. Please use common sense and listen to your body every step of the way.

We (the Wilen Sisters) are not medical authorities. The closest either of us comes is that Joan used to date a pharmacist and Lydia's favorite playwright is Doc Simon.

That brings us to an important point—this book being

SAFE. Our publisher did its part by having an M.D. who practices *integrative medicine* (see "Authors' Note") review all of the remedies in the book, and deem them "safe." Now you have to do your part by consulting with your health professional before starting any self-help health treatment.

Please, for your own well-being, heed the NOTES throughout the book. They stress the fact that our home-remedy suggestions are scientifically unproven and should not take the place of professional health care that may be needed for certain ailments and for persistent symptoms. Effective proven medical treatment is available for almost all conditions mentioned in this book. You can use the remedies in addition to, but not as a substitute for, professional help.

How do we know that the remedies work? It's as though our parents saw the future when they named us. Lydia is named after our mother's aunt, who was the town herbalist/midwife. Joan is named for our father's cousin, the town hypochondriac. It worked out great. As we researched and wrote each chapter, Joan would get symptoms—and we got the chance to try lots of remedies! The ones with which we don't have firsthand experience come highly recommended, usually by more than one source. We've reasoned it out: The remedies that work have been passed down from generation to generation, and the ones that didn't work most likely haven't survived the trip here.

While not all the remedies will be cure-alls for everyone, they're worth a try, and as Grandma used to say, "It wouldn't hurt!" (Actually, our grandmother used to say, "It vouldn't hoit!")

Since you seem to be interested in home remedies, we would love your input. Have you tried any of these remedies? What has been your experience with them?

Do you have any of your own remedies you would like to

share with us? We can be reached by mail at the address below.

Thank you for reading our book.

To your health!*

Joan Wilen and Lydia Wilen
P.O. Box 230416
Ansonia Station
New York, NY 10023-0416

*Gëzuar! (Albanian) Fi schettak! (Arabian) Genatzt! (Armenian) Prosit! (Austria) Op uw gezonheid! (Belgian) Naz dar! (Bohemian) Viva! (Brazilian) Yum sen! (Chinese) Na Zdravi! (Czechoslavakian) Skål! (Norwegian, Swedish, and Danish) Proost! (Dutch) Je zia sano! (Esperanto) Kippis! (Finnish) A votre santé! (French) Auf ihr wohol! (German) Eis Igian! (Greek) Kasûgta! (Greenlandic) Okole maluna! (Hawaiian) Kedves egeszsegere! (Hungarian) Santanka nu! (Icelandic) Jaikind! (Indian) Selamat! (Indonesian) Besalmati! (Iranian) A la salute! (Italian) Kampai! (Japanese) Kong gang ul wi ha yo! (Korean) I sveikas! (Lithuanian) Slamat minum! (Malayan) Salud! (Spanish) Saha wa'afiab! (Moroccan) Kia ora! (New Zealand) Zanda bashi (Pakistani) Mabuhay! (Philippine) Noroc! (Rumanian) Na zdorovia! (Russian) Sawasdi! (Thai) Serefe! (Turkish) Boovatje zdorovi! (Ukrainian) Iechyd da! (Welsh) Tsu gezunt! (Yiddish) Zivio! (Yugoslavian) Oogy wawa! (Zulu)

Preparation Guide

‡ BARLEY

Hippocrates, the father of medicine, felt that everyone should drink barley water daily to maintain good health. Barley is rich in iron and vitamin B. It is said to help prevent tooth decay and hair loss, improve fingernails and toenails, and help heal ulcers, diarrhea, and bronchial spasms.

Pearl or pearled barley has been milled. During the milling process, the double outer husk is removed, along with its nutrients. A less-refined version is pot or Scotch barley. Once it's gone through a less severe milling process, part of the bran layer remains, along with some of the nutrients. Hulled barley, with only the outer, inedible hull removed, is rich in dietary fiber, and has more iron, trace minerals, and four times the thiamine (B_1) than pearled barley. It's available at some health food stores, as is Scotch barley. If you can't get either, you will be able to get pearl barley at your supermarket.

BARLEY WATER: Boil 2 ounces of barley in 6 cups of water (distilled water if possible) until there's about half the water—3 cups—left in the pot. Strain. If necessary, add honey and lemon to taste.

‡ COCONUT MILK

To get to the milk in the easiest way possible, you need an ice pick or a screwdriver (Phillips is best), and a hammer. The coconut has three little black eyelike bald spots on it. Place the ice pick or screwdriver in the middle of one black spot, then hammer the end of it so that it pierces the coconut. Repeat the procedure with the other two black spots and then pour out the coconut milk. The hammer alone should then do the trick on the rest of the coconut. Always watch out for your fingers—but also watch your figure. Coconut meat is high in saturated fat.

‡ EYEWASH

Reminder: Always remove contact lenses before doing an eyewash.

You'll need an eye cup (available at drugstores). Carefully pour just-boiled water over the cup to clean it. Then, without contaminating the rim or inside surfaces of the cup, fill it half full with whichever eyewash you've selected. Apply the cup tightly to the eye to prevent spillage, then tilt your head backward. Open your eyelid wide and rotate your eyeball to thoroughly wash the eye. Use the same procedure with the other eye.

‡ GARLIC

When it comes to knowing about garlic, we wrote the book on it. We really did. It's appropriately called *Garlic— Nature's Super Healer* (Prentice Hall).

Garlic is a natural antibiotic with antiviral, antifungal, anticoagulant, and antiseptic properties. It can act as an expectorant and decongestant, antioxidant, germicide, anti-inflammatory agent, diuretic, sedative, and it is believed to contain cancer-preventive chemicals. It's also said to be an aphrodisiac—but if you reek of garlic, no one will come close enough to find out!

GARLIC JUICE: When a remedy calls for garlic juice, peel a clove of garlic, mince it finely onto a piece of cheesecloth, then squeeze the juice out of it. A garlic press will make the job easier.

‡ GINGER

Research herbalist Paul Schulick agrees with the name given to ginger in ancient India, *vishwabhesaj,* or the "universal medicine." Ginger earned the title because it's a profound anti-inflammatory, a strong antioxidant, an effective antimicrobial agent, the answer to a variety of digestive disorders, a natural therapy for menstrual discomfort, nausea, colds, parasites, morning sickness, motion sickness, and more. It also can be used as a daily tonic to increase general well-being.

GINGER TEA: Peel or scrub a nub of fresh ginger and cut it into three to five quarter-size pieces. Pour just-boiled water over it and let it steep for five to ten minutes. If you want strong ginger tea, *grate* a piece of ginger, then steep it, strain it and drink it. TV personality and chef Ainsley Harriott told us that he freezes ginger, which makes it easier to grate.

‡ HERB BATH

Beside offering a good relaxing time, the herbal bath can be extremely healing. The volatile oils of the herbs are activated by the heat of the water, which also opens your pores, allowing for absorption of the herbs. As you enjoy the bath, you're inhaling the herbs (aromatherapy), which pass through the nervous system to the brain, benefiting both mind and body.

HERB BATH DIRECTIONS: Simply take a handful of one or a combination of dried or fresh herbs and place them in the center of a white handkerchief. Secure the herbs in the handkerchief by turning it into a little knapsack. Toss the herb-filled knapsack into the tub and let the hot water fill the tub until it reaches the level you want it to be. When the water cools enough for you to sit comfortably, do so.

After your bath, open the handkerchief and spread the herbs out to dry. You can use them a couple of times more.

Instead of using dried or fresh herbs, you can use herbal essential oils. Oils cause the tub to be slippery. Be extra careful getting out of the tub, and be sure to clean the tub thoroughly after you've taken the bath.

‡ HERB TEA

Place a teaspoon of the herb, or the herb tea bag, in a glass or ceramic cup and pour just-boiled water over it. (The average water-to-herb ratio is 6 to 8 ounces of water to 1 round teaspoon of herb. There are exceptions, so be sure to read the directions on the herb tea package.)

According to the herb tea company Lion Cross, never use water that has been boiled before. The first boiling releases oxygen and the second boiling results in "flat," lifeless tea.

Cover the cup and let the tea steep for the amount of time suggested on the package. The general rule of thumb is: steep about three minutes for flowers and soft leaves; about five minutes for seeds and leaves; about ten minutes for hard seeds, roots, and barks. Of course, the longer the tea steeps, the stronger it gets.

Strain the tea, or remove the tea bag. If you need to sweeten it, use raw honey (never use sugar because it is said to negate the value of most herbs), and when it's cool enough, drink it slowly.

‡ ONION

The onion is in the same plant family as garlic and is almost as versatile. The ancient Egyptians looked at the onion as the symbol of the universe. It has been regarded as a universal healing food, used to treat earaches, colds, fever, wounds, diarrhea, insomnia, warts, and the list goes on. It is believed that a cut onion in a sickroom disinfects the air as it absorbs the germs in that room. Half an onion will help absorb the smell of a just-painted room. With that in mind, you may not want to use a cut piece of onion that has been in the kitchen for more than a day, unless you wrap it in plastic wrap and refrigerate it.

ONION JUICE: When a remedy calls for onion juice, grate an onion, put the gratings in a piece of cheesecloth, and squeeze out the juice.

‡ POMANDERS

To make an orange-spice pomander, you'll need:

1 thin-skinned orange
1 box of whole cloves
1 ounce orrisroot
1 ounce cinnamon
½ ounce nutmeg
2 feet of ¼″–½″ ribbon

Tie the ribbon around the orange and knot it, leaving two long ends of ribbon. Stick the cloves all over the orange, but not through the ribbon. Mix the three herbs together in a bowl, then place the orange in the bowl. Let it stay there for four or five days, turning the orange occasionally. At the end of that time, hang the orange-spice pomander in a closet.

‡ POTATOES

Raw, peeled, boiled, grated, and mashed potatoes; potato water; and potato poultices all help heal, according to American, English, and Irish folk medicine. In fact, a popular nineteenth-century Irish saying was, "Only two things in this world are too serious to be jested on: potatoes and matrimony."

The skin or peel of the potato is richer in fiber, iron, potassium, calcium, phosphorus, zinc, and C and B vitamins than the inside of the potato. Always leave the skin on when preparing potato water, but scrub it well.

Do not use potatoes that have a green tinge. The greenish coloring is a warning that there may be a high concentration of solanine, a toxic alkaloid that can affect nerve impulses and cause vomiting, cramps, and diarrhea. The same goes for potatoes that have started to sprout. They're a no-no.

POTATO WATER: Scrub 2 medium-size potatoes (use organic whenever possible) and cut them in half. Put the 4 halves in a pot with 4 cups of water (filtered, spring, or distilled, if possible) and bring to a boil. Lower the flame a little and let it cook for thirty minutes. Take out the potatoes (eating them is optional) and save the water. Most remedies say to drink 2 cups of potato water. Refrigerate the leftover water for next time.

‡ POULTICES

Poultices are usually made with vegetables, fruit, or herbs that are either minced, chopped, grated, crushed, mashed, and sometimes cooked. These ingredients are then wrapped in a clean fabric—cheesecloth, white cotton, unbleached muslin—and applied externally to the affected area.

A poultice is most effective when moist. When the poultice dries out, it should be changed—the cloth as well as the ingredients.

Whenever possible, use *fresh* fruits, vegetables, or herbs. If these are unavailable, then use dried herbs. To soften herbs, pour hot water over them. Do not let herbs steep in water that's still boiling, unless the remedy specifies to do it. Boiling most herbs will diminish their healing powers.

Let's use comfrey as an example of a typical poultice.

Cut a piece of cloth twice the size of the area it will

cover. If you're using a fresh leaf, wash it with cool water, then crush it in your hand. Place the leaf on one half of the cloth and fold over the other half. If you are making a poultice with dried comfrey root and leaves, pour hot water over the herb, then place the softened herb down the length of the cloth, about two inches from the edge. Roll the cloth around the herb so that it won't spill out and place it on the affected body part. Gently wrap an Ace bandage or another piece of cloth around the poultice to hold it in place and to keep in the moisture.

‡ SAUERKRAUT

Sauerkraut is fermented cabbage that has been a popular folk medicine throughout the world for centuries. Cabbage is a potent inhibitor of the human papilloma virus (HPV) that causes warts. The lactic acid in sauerkraut is said to encourage the growth of friendly bacteria and help destroy enemy bacteria in the large intestine (where many people believe disease may begin) and in other parts of the digestive tract. Sauerkraut is rich in vitamin B_6—which is important for brain and nervous system functions—and high in calcium—for healthy teeth and bones. In fact, in the hills of West Germany, it is reported that sauerkraut is used as a snack for children, to help prevent tooth decay, and heal bad skin conditions.

The sauerkraut that comes in cans has been processed, and the valuable properties may have been destroyed in the process. It is for that reason you should eat sauerkraut cold from the refrigerator, at room temperature, or after it's been warmed over a very low flame. Overheating may destroy the lactic acid and beneficial enzymes.

You can buy raw sauerkraut in jars in health food stores, or out of barrels in some ethnic stores. You can also make your own sauerkraut.

Ingredients and Supplies:

1 large head of white cabbage (about 8 cups when shredded)

8 teaspoons of sea salt

1 tablespoon of caraway seeds or fresh or dried dill (OPTIONAL)

1 large container (earthenware crock, glass bowl, or stainless steel cookware)

A cover or plate that fits snugly inside the above-mentioned container

A brick or stones or any 10-pound weight that's clean

A cloth or towel that will fit over the container

Preparation:

Remove the large loose outer leaves of the cabbage, rinse them, and leave them for later. Core and finely shred the rest of the cabbage. Spread a layer of cabbage (about 1 cup) on the bottom of the container. Sprinkle the layer with a teaspoon of sea salt and a few caraway seeds or dill. Repeat layering with cabbage, salt, and seeds, ending with a layer of salt. Place those loose outer leaves of cabbage over the top layer. Then, press the cabbage down with the plate or cover and place the weight on top of it. Cover the entire container with a cloth or towel and set it aside in a warm place for seven to twelve days, depending on how strong you like your sauerkraut.

After a week or more, remove the weight and the plate. Throw away the leaves on top and skim off the yucky-looking mold from the top layer. Transfer the sauerkraut from the container to glass jars with lids, and refrigerate. It should keep for about a month.

Remedies

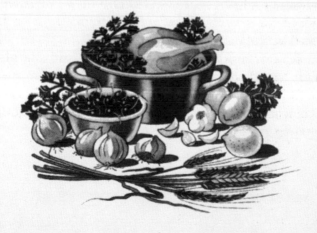

‡Alcoholism

Drinking in excess can make you look wrinkled and haggard, can destroy vital organs and, in general, ruin your life. We know someone who read so much about the bad effects of drinking that he gave up reading.

But seriously . . . For the problem drinker, we strongly recommend the leading self-help organization for combating alcoholism: Alcoholics Anonymous. Check the white pages of the telephone book for your local chapter.

This section deals with the social drinker who, occasionally, has one too many.

‡ SOBERING UP

The following remedies can help sober people up—that is, make them more alert and communicative. However, *do not trust or depend on those people's reflexes*, especially behind the wheel of a car.

To start with, if a drunk person imagines that the room is spinning, have him or her lie down on a bed and put one foot on the floor to stop that feeling.

To help sober up an intoxicated person, try feeding him or her cucumber—as much as he or she is willing to eat.

The cuke's enzyme, erepsin, may dramatically lessen the effect of alcohol.

Honey contains fructose, which promotes the chemical breakdown of alcohol. If you know that the drunk person is *not* allergic to honey and is not a diabetic, give him or her 1 or 2 teaspoons of honey. Follow that up with 1 teaspoon of it every half hour for the next couple of hours.

Try sobering up someone who's tipsy by massaging the tip of his or her nose.

CAUTION: Stimulation of the tip of the nose can cause vomiting, so don't stand right in front of the person you're sobering up.

‡ HANGOVERS

Hangovers can be caused by an allergy or sensitivity to something you drank. Put 1 drop of that drink in a glass of water. Take three sips of it. If the hangover symptoms do not disappear within five minutes, then drink the rest of the glass of water. If you still don't feel better within a few minutes, then your hangover is not allergy-caused. Try some other remedy.

For the morning after the night before, take ⅛ teaspoon of cayenne pepper in a glass of water.

Evening primrose oil (soft gels available at health food stores) is said to help replenish the amino acids and gamma-linoleic acid that's lost when you drink alcoholic beverages. Take 1,000 mg with lots of water or orange juice before you zonk out. Too late for that? Okay then, take it when you wake up and are desperate for anything that will help you feel human again.

According to the Chinese, a cup of ginger tea (see "Preparation Guide") will help settle an unsettled stomach caused by a hangover. To relieve eye, ear, mouth, nose, and brain pain from the hangover, they recommend kneading the fleshy part of the hand between the thumb and the index finger on both hands. For the pounding hangover headache, massage each thumb, just below the knuckles.

Take 1 tablespoon of honey every minute for five minutes. Repeat the procedure one half hour later.

Rub ¼ lemon on each armpit. That may ease the discomfort of a hangover.

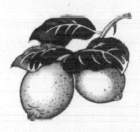

‡ MORNING-AFTER BREAKFAST
Banana and milk is the breakfast of choice of many hangover sufferers. It may be effective due to the fact that alcohol depletes the magnesium in one's body, and bananas and milk replenish the supply.

You may want to add to that: tomato, carrot, celery and/or beet juice to replenish the B and C vitamins along with some trace minerals that alcohol may also deplete.

Naturalist and writer Pliny the Elder recommended eating the eggs of an owl. While they may be hard to come by, all eggs are a source of cysteine, which helps the body manufacture glutathione, an antioxidant that gets depleted when alcohol is present. So an omelet could be a helpful hangover breakfast. Pliny may have eased the symptoms of many a hangover with those eggs. Look who was the wise old owl, after all. . . .

NOTE: If you really need to recover rapidly from a hangover, go to your local doctor, dentist, or hospital, and, under medical supervision, take ten snorts of oxygen.

‡Arthritis (Rheumatism, Bursitis, Gout), Muscle Aches, Pains, and Sprains

One authority in the field feels that arthritis is a catchall term that includes rheumatism, bursitis, and gout. Another specialist believes that arthritis is a form of rheumatism. Still another claims there is no such ailment as rheumatism, that it's a term for several diseases, including arthritis.

No matter what it's called, everyone agrees on two things: Oh, the pain! and that all these conditions (herein bunched under the heading of "Arthritis") involve inflammation of connective tissue of one or more joints.

Knowledge is power! Check your local library, the Internet, and our suggested reading list for books on arthritis (and there are lots of them). Learn about nonchemical treatments and low-acid diets. There are foods that have been classified as nightshade foods—white potatoes, eggplants, green peppers, and tomatoes being the most common ones—that may contribute to the pain of some arthritis sufferers. Consider being professionally tested for a sensitivity to the nightshade foods. Work with a health professional to evaluate your condition and to help you find safe, sensible methods of treatment for relief.

Here are remedies that have been said to be successful for many arthritis sufferers—that is, *former* arthritis sufferers. Note: These remedies may not be substitutions for professional medical treatment.

‡ ARTHRITIS

Cherries are said to be effective because they seem to help prevent crystallization of uric acid and to reduce the uric acid levels in the blood. It is also said that cherries have been known to help the arthritic bumps on knuckles disappear.

EAT CHERRIES! Any kind—sweet or sour, fresh, canned or frozen, black, Royal Anne or Bing. DRINK CHERRY JUICE! Available without preservatives or sugar added, and also in a concentrated form at health food stores.

One source says to eat cherries and drink the juice throughout the day for four days, then stop for four days and then start all over again. Another source says to eat up to a dozen cherries a day in addition to drinking a glass of cherry juice. Find a happy medium by using your own good judgment as to cherry dosage. Listen to your body. You'll know soon enough if the cherries seem to be making you feel better.

Eat a portion of fresh string beans every day, or juice the string beans and drink a glassful daily. String beans contain vitamins A, B_1, B_2, and C and supposedly help overly acid conditions such as arthritis.

Steep 1 cup of fully packed parsley in 1 quart of boiling water. After fifteen minutes, strain and refrigerate.

DOSE: ½ cup before breakfast, ½ cup before dinner, and ½ cup anytime pain is particularly severe.

Garlic has been used to quiet arthritis pain quickly. Rub a freshly cut clove of garlic on painful areas. Also, take a garlic supplement—after breakfast and after dinner.

Grate 3 tablespoons of horseradish and stir it into ½ cup of boiled milk. Pour the mixture onto a piece of cheesecloth, then apply it to the painful area. By the time the poultice cools, you may have some relief.

Celery contains many nourishing salts and organic sulfur. Some modern herbalists believe that celery has the power to help neutralize uric acid and other excess acids in the body. Eat fresh celery daily. The leaves on top of celery stalks are also good to eat. If the roughage is rough on your digestive system, place the tops and tough parts of the stalk in a nonaluminum pan. Cover with water and slowly bring to a boil. Then simmer for ten to fifteen minutes. Strain and pour into a jar.

DOSE: Drink 8 ounces three times a day, one half hour before each meal.

You can vary your celery intake by drinking celery seed tea and/or juiced celery stalks, or do as the Rumanians do and cook celery in milk. Remember, celery is a diuretic, so plan your day accordingly.

According to results published in *The Journal of the American Medical Association*, based on experiments by a study team at the Brusch Medical Center in Massachusetts, cod-liver oil in milk helped to reduce cholesterol levels, improve blood chemistry and complexion, increase energy, and correct stomach problems, blood sugar balance, blood pressure, and tissue inflammation.

Mix 1 tablespoon of cod-liver oil (emulsified Norwegian cod-liver oil is nonfishy) in 6 ounces of milk.

DOSE: Drink it on an empty stomach, one half hour before breakfast and one half hour before dinner.

NOTE: Cod-liver oil is a source of vitamins A and D. If you are taking A and D supplements, check the dosages carefully. The daily recommended dosage of vitamin A is 10,000 IU, for vitamin D 400 IU. DO NOT EXCEED THOSE AMOUNTS WITHOUT THE SUPERVISION OF A HEALTH PROFESSIONAL.

Applying cod-liver oil externally is said to help relieve the popping noises of the joints.

Even if you have a sensitivity to nightshade foods, external potato remedies can be used, as they have been for centuries. Carry a raw potato in your pocket. Don't leave home without it! When it shrivels up after a day or two, replace it with a fresh potato. It supposedly draws out the poisons and acids that might be causing the problem and pain.

For dealing with the affected areas more directly, dice 2 cups of unpeeled potatoes and put them in a nonaluminum saucepan with 5 cups of water. Boil gently until about half the water is left. While the water is hot, but not scalding, dunk a clean cloth in the potato water, wring it out and apply it to the painful parts of the body. Repeat the procedure for as long as your patience holds out, or the pain persists—whichever goes first.

When you're feeling twinges in the hinges all over your body, take a bath in rose petals. Use petals from three or four roses that are about to wither and throw them in your bathwater. It should give you a rosy outlook.

Temporary Relief for Women Only: Arthritic pains often disappear when a woman is pregnant. As soon as researchers find the reason for this, they may also find a permanent cure.

Eating strawberries and very little else for a few days is said to be a possible cure for gout. Strawberries are a powerful alkalizer and contain calcium, iron, and an ingredient known as salacin, which soothes inflammatory conditions. It worked so well for botanist Linnaeus that he referred to strawberries as "a blessing of the gods."

Apple cider vinegar has been used in various ways to help arthritis sufferers. See which of the following remedies is most palatable and convenient for you. Don't forget to have patience and give it at least three weeks to work.

Every morning and every evening, take 1 teaspoon of honey mixed with 1 teaspoon of apple cider vinegar. Or: Before each meal (three times a day), drink a glass of water containing 2 teaspoons of apple cider vinegar. Or: Between lunch and dinner, drink a mixture of 2 ounces of apple cider vinegar added to 6 ounces of water. Drink it down slowly.

Prepare a poultice of coarse (kosher) salt that has been heated in a frying pan. Then apply it to the painful area. To keep the salt comfortably warm, put a hot water bottle on top of it. (Chances are, this old home remedy draws out the pain effectively with nonkosher salt, too.)

‡ CHARLEY HORSE (MUSCLE STIFFNESS)

Prepare strong ginger tea with 2 teaspoons of ginger powder or fresh, grated ginger root in 2 cups of water. Let it simmer until the water turns yellowish in color. Add the ginger tea to a bathful of warm water. Relax in the tub for twenty to thirty minutes. This ginger tea bath may relieve muscle stiffness and soreness and is wonderful for one's circulation.

Soak in a tub of "old faithful"—Epsom salts. Pour 3 cupsful of it in warm water. Stay in the water twenty to thirty minutes and your charley horse pain may start to ease.

‡ SPRAINS

During the first twelve hours after the injury, starting as soon as possible, apply an ice-cold water compress to the area to reduce the swelling caused by the sprain. Leave the compress on for twenty minutes, then take it off for twenty minutes. Extend the twelve hours of cold compresses to twenty-four hours if necessary. It would be wise to seek medical attention to make sure the sprain is nothing more than a sprain and not a fractured, chipped, or dislocated bone.

To help relieve the pain from a severe sprain, rub on leek liniment. To prepare the liniment, simmer 4 leeks in boiling water until they're mushy. Pour off the water and mash 4 tablespoons of coconut butter into the leek. As soon as it's cool, massage it into the sprained area. Keep the remaining liniment in a covered container. It can also be used for most muscle aches and pains.

‡Asthma

During an asthma attack, bronchial tubes narrow and secrete an excess of mucus, making it very hard to breathe.

Asthma in certain people may be attributed to allergies or emotional problems, or possibly a combination of both.

In the 1800s, Peter Latham said, "You cannot be sure of the success of your remedy, while you are still uncertain of the nature of the disease." And so it is with asthma.

Folk medicine legends abound with curious asthma remedies from around the world:

European and Australian folklore advocates swallowing a handful of spiderwebs rolled into a ball. Deep in the heart of Texas, they are said to sleep on the uncleaned wool of recently sheared sheep. The asthma is, legend has it, absorbed by the wool. Another old Texas home remedy requires the asthmatic to get a chihuahua (Mexican hairless dog). The theory is that the asthma goes from the patient to the dog, but the dog does not suffer from it. According to Kentucky folklore, wearing a string of amber beads around the neck may cure asthma. With the cost of a full strand of amber these days, it would be cheaper to buy a chihuahua, have him get asthma, then buy that tiny dog a strand of amber.

These legendary folk remedies make for good conversation, but in the midst of an asthma attack, who can talk?

The remedies we recommend for asthmatic conditions are more practical and easier to come by than those listed above.

While trying to find the most effective asthma-relieving remedy, it's important that you consult with a health professional every step of the way. These remedies are not substitutes for professional medical treatment.

Eat 3 to 6 apricots a day. They may help promote healing of lung and bronchial conditions.

Jerusalem artichokes, eaten daily, may be a real plus for nourishing the lungs of the asthmatic. (See "Diabetes" for more details on these terrific tubers.)

Put 4 cups of sunflower seeds in 2 quarts of water and boil it down to 1 quart of water. Strain out the little pieces of sunflower seeds, then add 1 pint of honey and boil it down to a syrupy consistency.
DOSE: 1 teaspoon one half hour after each meal.

A relative told us that in the "old country," a remedy used at the onset of an asthma attack was to inhale the steam from boiling potatoes that were cut in pieces with the skin left on them. With or without the potatoes, inhaling steam can be beneficial. Be careful: Steam is powerful and can burn the skin.

Mix 1 teaspoon of grated horseradish with 1 teaspoon of honey and take it every night before bedtime.

Slice 2 large raw onions into a jar. Pour 2 cups of honey over it. Close the jar and let it stand overnight. Next morning you're ready to start taking the "honion" syrup.
DOSE: 1 teaspoon one half hour after each meal and 1 teaspoon before bed.

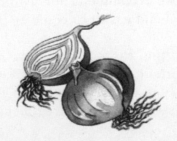

Similar to but more potent than the sunflower seed syrup described earlier in this chapter is this garlic syrup. Separate and peel the cloves of 3 entire garlic bulbs. Simmer them in a nonaluminum pan with 2 cups of water. When the garlic cloves are soft and there's about a cup of water left in the pan, remove the garlic and put it in a jar. Then, add 1 cup of cider vinegar and ¼ cup of honey to the water that's left in the pan, boiling the mixture until it's syrupy. Pour the syrup over the garlic in the jar. Cover the jar and let it stand overnight.

DOSE: 1 or 2 cloves of garlic with a teaspoon of syrup every morning on an empty stomach.

Buy either concentrated cranberry juice, sold at health food stores, or unconcentrated cranberry juice, sold at most supermarkets (READ THE INGREDIENTS ON THE LABEL and make sure there are no preservatives or sugar added), or make your own with 1 pound of cranberries in 1 pint of water. Boil until the cranberries are very mushy. Then, pour the mixture into a jar and keep it in the refrigerator.

DOSE: Drink 2 tablespoons one half hour before each meal and at the onset of an asthma attack.

‡Blood

Blood is an extremely complex substance consisting of many liquid and solid elements including red and white blood cells, blood platelets, and blood plasma.

The average adult has between 5 and 6 quarts of blood circulating through the body by way of the blood vessels.

To help circulation as well as purification of the blood and aid in elimination of iron-deficiency anemia, we offer suggestions *with* the suggestion you *first* have appropriate professional blood tests and consult with a physician *before* embarking on any self-help program.

‡ BLOOD TEST ACCURACY

To discover cholesterol levels, red blood cell counts, and a long list of other important physical data, blood tests are required. The standards for most of those tests were established among people *who were standing* when their blood was drawn. According to a report in *Lancet*, when you stand, gravity pushes fluid from your blood into surrounding tissues. If blood were to be taken when a person is lying down, there would be a marked difference in the results from the blood that was taken when that same person was standing. That difference can mean misdiagnoses, and even mistreatment. Every time blood is drawn, always stay in the same position, preferably standing.

‡ IRON-DEFICIENCY ANEMIA

Grape juice (no sugar or preservatives added) is a wonderful source of iron. Drink 8 ounces every day.

Eat raw spinach salads often. Be sure to wash the spinach thoroughly. Combine any of the following in your spinach salad: watercress, radish, kohlrabi, garlic, chives, leek, and onion. They're all high in iron.

Every morning after breakfast and every evening after dinner, eat 2 dried apricots.

Snack on raisins.

NOTE: In the case of a serious iron deficiency, you may require more iron than you can possibly get from any or all of the ideas above. We suggest you seek help from a health professional.

‡ BLOOD FORTIFIERS

Raw (not canned) sauerkraut is said to do a super job of fortifying the blood. It also helps rejuvenate the body in other ways. Eat 2 to 4 tablespoons a day, right after a meal. (Raw sauerkraut can be found at health food stores, or see "Preparation Guide" and learn to prepare your own sauerkraut.)

CHECK WITH YOUR MEDICAL ADVISER BEFORE GOING ON THIS ONE-DAY FAST. Combine 2 tablespoons of lemon, 1 tablespoon of honey, and a cup of warm water.
DOSE: Every two hours, from morning until two hours before bedtime, take 2 tablespoons of the mixture. No food throughout the day, just the lemon/honey/water mixture.

Raw (not cooked or canned) pumpkin pulp and squash are said to have purifying properties. Eat them in salads.

When they're in season, a peach a day helps wash toxins away.

Garlic is said to help thin and fortify the blood. Eat raw garlic and/or take garlic supplements daily.

Drink fresh carrot juice as often as once a day if you have access to a juicer, or eat raw carrots. They contain calcium, potassium, phosphorus, and vitamins A, B_1, B_2, and C.

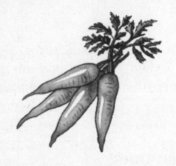

‡ CIRCULATION

Once a day, mix ⅛ teaspoon of cayenne pepper in a cup of water and drink it down. It's not easy to take, but it may be beneficial to the circulatory system, since cayenne pepper is reputed to be the purest herbal stimulant.

Japanese medicine recommends ginger footbaths to improve circulation. Add a cup of fresh, minced ginger to a basin with 2 quarts of warm water, or divide the water and ginger into two plastic shoe boxes. Soak your feet in the water until they're rosy red. Then, dry thoroughly and notice a more energized feeling.

‡ VARICOSE VEINS

Heed these simple suggestions to keep varicose veins from getting worse:

- Keep your feet elevated as much as possible. It's ideal to elevate your legs at or above the level of your heart for twenty minutes a few times a day.
- Never sit with your legs crossed.
- Don't wear knee-high stockings or tight socks.
- Wear flats or very low heels, not high heels.
- If you're overweight, do your legs a favor and lose those extra pounds.
- Exercise. Just walking a half hour every day will help with circulation.

Here are some suggestions that may help improve the condition of your varicose veins: Take 1 bilberry capsule (80 mg) with each meal and 1 bromelain capsule (500 to 1,000 mg) with each meal. Once a day, take a capsule (150 mg) of butcher's broom. All are available at health food stores. These herbs do wonderful things, including helping your circulation, and helping the walls of your veins maintain their shape.

Reduce the swelling and constriction of varicose veins by wrapping a cheesecloth bandage soaked in witch hazel around the affected area. Lie down, raise your legs, and relax.

At the end of every day, stand in a tub of cold water up to the knees. After two or three minutes, dry the legs with a coarse towel, then walk around your home at a brisk pace, also for about two to three minutes.

Take horse chestnut capsules, 300 mg (available at health food stores), once or twice a day.

‡Blood Pressure

The most important dietary recommendation for lowering blood pressure, according to Jade Beutler, licensed health care practitioner, is to increase the consumption of plant foods in the diet. A primarily vegetarian diet typically contains less saturated fat and refined carbohydrates, and more potassium, complex carbohydrates, fiber, calcium, magnesium, vitamin C, and essential fatty acids.

Double-blind studies have demonstrated that either fish oil supplements or flaxseed oil, both rich in omega-3 oils, are very effective in lowering blood pressure. (See "And Now May We Prevent . . ." for detailed *flaxseed oil* information.)

When blood pressure is measured, there are two numbers reported: the first and higher number is the systolic. It measures the pressure inside the arteries the second the heart beats. The diastolic is the lower number and measures the pressure in the arteries when the heart is at rest.

More than twenty million Americans have high blood pressure (hypertension). If you're one of those people, you are not alone.

You probably already know the following basics. Hopefully, you'll take a look at your lifestyle and, once and for all, do something about it!

• If you're overweight, diet sensibly (without diet pills). Eliminate salt and cut down or cut out meat.
• To reduce the stress from your everyday life, try biofeedback and/or meditation. Ask a health professional for guidance and reputable contacts.
• If you smoke, stop!
• If you drink, stop! or at least cut down drastically.

Read on for additional high and low blood pressure health hints.

‡ HIGH BLOOD PRESSURE

Eat 2 apples a day. The pectin in apples may help lower high blood pressure.

Eat raw garlic in salads and use it in cooking. Also take garlic supplements daily—one after breakfast and one after dinner.

According to a university study, blood pressure can be reduced by staring at fish in a fish tank. The relaxation benefits of fish-watching are equal to biofeedback and meditation. If caring for a tank of fish isn't for you, check the Internet or your local video store for tapes of aquariums and fish swimming in their natural habitats.

Cucumbers are rich in potassium, phosphorus, and calcium. They're also a good diuretic and calming agent. To help bring down blood pressure, try eating a cucumber every day. If you have a juicer, drink ½ cup of fresh cucumber juice. You can also include some carrots and parsley, which is another good diuretic, in the juice.

Drink 2 cups of potato water daily. (See "Preparation Guide.")

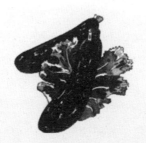

‡ BLOOD PRESSURE STABILIZERS

Just as there are people with high blood pressure, there are people (not as many) with low blood pressure. The following remedy is said to be a blood pressure regulator and stabilizer:

Scientific studies have shown that five to ten minutes of laughter first thing in the morning improves blood pressure levels. The problem is, what's there to laugh at first thing in the morning? There's usually a funny local disc jockey on radio, or go on-line and type in "jokes" at any Internet search engine (Yahoo, Alta Vista, Dogpile, Excite).

‡Burns

Burns are classified by degrees. A first-degree burn involves painful, red, unbroken skin. A second-degree burn involves painful blisters and broken skin. A third-degree burn destroys underlying tissue as well as surface skin. It may be painless because nerve endings may have also been destroyed. A fourth-degree burn involves deeply charred and blackened areas of the skin.

Second-degree burns that cover an extensive area of skin and *all* third- and fourth-degree burns require immediate medical attention. Any kind of burn on the face should also receive immediate medical attention as a precaution against swollen breathing passages.

As for first-degree burns—grabbing a hot pot handle, grasping the iron side of an iron, the oven door closing on your forearm, a splattering of boiling oil—here are first-aid suggestions for these burns, using mostly handy household items, that is, with the exception of cow dung and mud. Then again, if you're "home on the range," those *are* the handy household items.

‡ FIRST-DEGREE BURNS
Apply cold water or cold compresses first! Then:

Draw out the heat and pain by applying a slice of raw potato, or a piece of fresh pumpkin pulp, or a slice of raw onion. Leave the potato, pumpkin or onion on the burn for fifteen minutes, off for five minutes and then put a fresh piece on for another fifteen minutes.

If you burn yourself while baking and happen to have salt-free unbaked pie crust around, roll it thin and place it on the entire surface of the burn. Let it stay on until it dries up and falls off by itself.

If you have vitamin E or garlic oil capsules, puncture either one of them and squeeze the contents directly on the burn.

Uncooked chicken fat placed directly on burns and scalds is said to be quite soothing.

If you have a smooth piece of charcoal, put it on the burn and keep it there for an hour. Within minutes, the pain may begin to subside.

Make a poultice of raw sauerkraut and apply it to the burned area. If you don't have sauerkraut, use crushed comfrey root with a little honey. In fact, just plain honey on the burn may ease the pain and help the healing process.

If you're outdoors, pack mud on the burn to draw out the heat.

Spread apple butter over the burned area. As it dries, add another coat to it. Keep adding coats for a day or two, until the burn is just about butter—uh, better.

People have had remarkable results with apple cider vinegar. Pour it on the burned or scalded area.

Keep an aloe vera plant in your home. It's like growing a tube of ointment. Break off about a ½-inch piece of stem. Squeeze it so that the juice oozes out onto the burned area. The juice is most effective if the plant is at least two to three years old and the stems have little bumps on the edges.

‡ SECOND-DEGREE BURNS

For *at least* a half hour, dip the burned area in cold water, or apply a towel that's been drenched in ice-cold water. DO NOT USE LARD, BUTTER, OR A SALVE ON THE BURN! They seal in the heat, and when you get medical attention, the doctor has to wipe off the goo to see the condition of the skin.

If the burn is on an arm or leg, keep the limb raised in the air to help prevent swelling.

‡ CHEMICAL AND ACID BURNS

Until you get medical attention, immediately get the affected area under the closest running water—a sink, a garden hose, or the shower. The running water will help wash the chemicals off the skin. Keep the water running on the burned skin for at least twenty minutes or until medical help arrives.

‡ BURNED TONGUE

Keep rinsing mouth with cold water. A few drops of vanilla extract may relieve the pain.

‡ SUNBURN

When you've gotten more than you've basked for, fill a quart jar with equal parts of milk and ice and 2 tablespoons of salt. Soak a washcloth in the mixture and place it on the sunburned area. Leave it on for about fifteen minutes. Repeat the procedure three to four times throughout the day.

Steep 6 regular (nonherbal) tea bags in a quart of hot water. When the tea is strong and cool, drench a washcloth in the liquid and apply it to the sunburned area. Repeat the procedure until you get relief.

Spread yogurt or sour cream over the sunburned area, particularly the face. Leave it on for twenty minutes, then rinse off with lukewarm water. The yogurt or sour cream is said to take the heat out of the sunburn and tighten pores, too.

NOTE: Severe sunburns can be second-degree burns. If sunburned skin is broken or blistering, treatment should include cold water followed by a dry (preferably sterile) dressing.

‡ SUNBURNED EYES
Make a poultice of grated apples and rest it on your closed eyelids for a relaxing hour.

Make a poultice from the lightly beaten white of an egg. Bandage the poultice on the closed eyes and leave it there overnight. Chances are there will be a big improvement next morning.

Take vitamin C—500 mg—twice a day to help take out the burn.

‡Colds, Etc.

If you're out there with a red, runny nose, chest congestion, and that achy flu feeling, instead of making much achoo about nothing, keep reading for some simple cold-helping hints.

‡ COLDS/FLU

The first round of ammunition for fighting the cold war is chicken soup (Jewish penicillin). According to *Medical World News*, the director of medical services at Mount Sinai Medical Center in Miami Beach, Dr. Marvin A. Sackner, proved that chicken soup can help cure a cold.

Using a bronchofiberscope and cineroentgenograms and measurements of mucous velocity, Dr. Sackner tested the effectiveness of hot chicken soup and hot and cold water. Cold water lowered nasal clearance. Hot water improved it, but it was nothing compared to the improvement after hot chicken soup. Then, to negate the effects of the steam from the hot water and hot chicken soup, the fluids were sipped through straws from covered containers. Hot water had very little effect this way. The hot chicken soup still had some benefit.

CHICKEN SOUP RECIPE:
4–5 pounds of chicken parts
3 carrots, scrubbed or peeled, cut in thirds

2 parsnips, scrubbed, cut in thirds
2 celery stalks with leaves, cut in thirds
1 large onion cut in half
1 green pepper, cut in half and cleaned out
10 cups of water
1 to 2 teaspoons of salt
2 sprigs dill (optional), or ½ teaspoon of dill seeds
4 parsley sprigs
4 cloves of garlic, crushed

Add the chicken, carrots, parsnips, celery, onion, green pepper, water, and salt to a big pot. Wrap the dill or dill seeds, parsley, and garlic in cheesecloth and add that to the pot. Bring it to a boil, clean off the scum from the top of the soup, cover, and simmer for two and a half to three hours. Remove the chicken and the vegetables. Refrigerate the soup overnight. Next day, before heating the soup, remove the top layer of fat, skimming the surface with a spoon. Add the chicken and vegetables, heat and— Eat! Eat! Before it gets cold!

In the USSR, garlic is known as Russian penicillin. It has been reported that colds have actually disappeared within hours—a day at most—after taking garlic. Keep a peeled clove of garlic in the mouth, between the cheek and teeth. Do not chew it. Occasionally, release a little garlic juice by digging the teeth into the clove. Replace the clove every three to four hours.

The allicin in garlic is an excellent mucus-thinner and bacteria-killer. It's no wonder many cold remedies include garlic.

If taking garlic by mouth is not for you, then peel and crush 6 cloves of garlic. Mix them into ½ cup of white lard or vegetable shortening. Spread the mush on the soles of the feet and cover them with a (preferably warmed) towel or flannel cloth. Put plastic wrap under the feet to protect the bedding. Garlic is so powerful that even though it's applied to one's feet, it will be on one's breath, too.

Apply a fresh batch of the mixture every five hours until the cold is gone.

Prepare tea by steeping equal parts of cinnamon, sage, and bay leaves in hot water. Strain, and before drinking the tea, add 1 tablespoon of lemon juice. If necessary, sweeten with honey.

Keep flushing out your system by drinking lots of non-dairy liquids—unsweetened fruit juices, herbal tea (see above), and just plain water.

When our friend, the contessa from the Italian hills, has a cold, she makes a mug of very strong, regular tea and adds 1 tablespoon of honey, 1 tablespoon of cognac, 1 teaspoon of butter, and ¼ teaspoon of cinnamon. She drinks it as hot as she can and goes to bed between cotton sheets. If she wakes up during the night and is all sweaty, she changes her bedclothes and sheets and goes back to bed. By morning, she feels *molto bene!*

People have been known to fake a cold just to take this: Combine 4 teaspoons of rum with the juice of 1 lemon and 3 teaspoons of honey. Then add it to a glass of hot water and drink it before retiring. And don't tell us you plan to retire in another fourteen years.

Mix ¼ cup of apple cider vinegar with an equal amount of honey. It's an elixir that is particularly effective for a cold with a sore throat.
DOSE: Take 1 tablespoon six to eight times a day.

Boil down ½ cup of sunflower seeds (without the shells, of course) in 5 cups of water until there's about 2 cups of liquid left in the pot. Then stir in ¼ cup of honey and ¾ cup of gin. This potion is particularly good for chest colds.

DOSE: Take 2 teaspoons three times a day at mealtime.

Mix the white of 1 raw egg with 4 teaspoons of prepared mustard and rub it on the chest. Take a (preferably white) towel and dip it in hot water, then wring it out and place it on top of the mixture already on the chest. As soon as the towel is cool, redip it in hot water, wring it out, and again put it back on the chest. Reapply the towel four or five times. After the last application of the towel, wash off the chest, dry thoroughly, bundle up, and go to bed.

To stimulate appropriate acupuncture points that can help a cold, place an ice cube on the bottom of both big toes. Keep them in place with an Ace bandage or piece of cloth. Place feet in a basin, or in two plastic shoe boxes, or on plastic to avoid a mess from the melting ice. Do this procedure morning, noon, and night.

‡ SWEAT-IT-OUT DRINK

"What doesn't kill you, will make you stronger." That's the way we felt about the drink our grandmother (Bubbie) made the second someone in our family came down with a cold. The dreaded drink was called a *guggle-muggle*. We thought it was a cute name that Bubbie made up. Imagine our surprise when Edward Koch, during his last term in office as mayor of New York, talked about an ancient cure: his family's recipe for a *guggle-muggle*.

It seems that many Jewish families have their own *guggle-muggle* recipes—some more palatable than others. Our family's is the worst; Mr. Koch's is one of the best. As Ed Koch said, "It is not only medically superb, it is delicious!" And, with his permission, we share with you the Koch family for-adults-only *guggle-muggle* recipe:

In a saucepan, add the juice of 1 grapefruit, 1 lemon, 1 orange (preferably a Temple orange, because of its taste and the appropriateness of its name), and 1 tablespoon of honey. Bring it to a boil while stirring. Take it off the fire, pour it into a glass, then add at least 1 ounce of your favorite liquor. (Brandy is Ed Koch's.) As with most *guggle-muggles*, drink it down, then get under the covers and go to sleep. Next morning, no cold.

‡ FEVER

Bind sliced onions or peeled garlic cloves to the bottoms of the feet. Don't be surprised if it gives you onion or garlic breath. And don't be surprised if it brings down your temperature.

Eat grapes (in season) throughout the day. Also, dilute pure grape juice and sip some of it throughout the day. Drink it at room temperature, never chilled.

Boil 4 cups (1 quart) of water with ½ teaspoon of cayenne pepper. As you're ready to drink each of these 4 cups throughout the day, add to each cup 1 teaspoon of honey and ¼ cup of orange juice. Heat it up just a little and then drink it slowly.

‡ SINUS

Slowly, cautiously, and gently inhale the vapors of freshly grated horseradish (known in certain circles as the Jewish Dristan). While you're at it, mix grated horseradish with lemon juice (equal amounts of each).

DOSE: Eat 1 teaspoon one full hour before breakfast and

at least one hour after dinner. It gives long-lasting relief to some sinus sufferers who are good about taking it every day without fail.

Crush 1 clove of garlic into ¼ cup of water. Sip up the garlicky water into an eyedropper. (Make sure no pieces get into the dropper.)

DOSE: 10 drops of clear garlic water per nostril, three times a day for three days. At the end of the three days, there should be a noticeable clearing up of the sinus infection.

Buy garlic pills and parsley pills.

DOSE: Take 2 garlic pills and 2 parsley pills every four hours that you're awake. (That should add up to four times a day.) At the end of six days, you should be breathing a lot easier.

To stop sniffling, swallow 1 teaspoon of honey with freshly ground pepper sprinkled on it. Don't inhale the pepper or you'll get rid of the sniffles and start sneezing.

‡ HAY FEVER

Chew a bite-size chunk of honeycomb at the start of a hay fever attack. The honey is delicious. The comb part turns into a ball of wax that should be chewed for ten to fifteen minutes. Our experience has been that it gives temporary relief from a hay fever attack.

The U.S. Army tested honeycomb as a desensitizing and antiallergenic substance for hay fever. Their results were very encouraging, especially those from patients who chewed the honeycomb. (After chewing the waxy stuff, throw it out rather than swallow it.)

(See "And Now May We Prevent . . ." for immunizing against hay fever.)

Several studies have shown that bioflavonoids help the body utilize vitamin C more effectively.

After the morning and evening meals, take 1 pantothenic acid (50 mg) and 1 vitamin C (500 mg) tablet along with a bioflavonoid—a grapefruit, orange, a few strawberries, grapes or prunes. If you don't want a fruit, take a teaspoon of grated orange or lemon peel sweetened with a little honey. This remedy has been said to have brought relief to many hay fever sufferers.

‡ NOSEBLEEDS

When you have a nosebleed, sit or stand. Do not lie down. Do not put your head back. It will cause you to swallow blood.

NOTE: Nasal hemorrhaging—blood flowing from both nostrils—requires immediate medical attention. Rush to the nearest doctor or hospital emergency room.

Also, recurrent nosebleeds may be a symptom of an underlying ailment. Seek appropriate medical attention.

For the occasional nosebleed, the first thing to do is to gently blow your nose. It may help rid your nostril of blood clots that may prevent a blood vessel from sealing. Then try any of the following remedies:

When one of us had a nosebleed, our father would take a half-dollar, put it on the frozen ice cube tray for a few seconds, then press it to the back of the sufferer's neck. We looked forward to getting nosebleeds, since we would get to keep the half-dollar. Ice at the nape of the neck has also been known to work, as has raw onion, but neither is as profitable.

Nosebleeds have been known to stop when you immerse your hands in warm water. Get a nosebleed . . . do the dishes!

Take your thumb and forefinger and pinch your nose right below the hard, bony part—about halfway down the nose. Stay that way for seven minutes, and you should no longer have a nosebleed.

Fold a small piece of brown grocery-bag paper and place it between the upper lip and the gum. It's been known to stop a bloody nose in no time.

‡Constipation and Regularity

You are most likely reading this page because you're seeking a natural laxative. Therefore, you may already know that the commercial chemical laxatives can kill friendly bacteria, can lessen the absorption of nutrients, can stuff up the intestinal walls, can turn users into addicts, can get rid of necessary vitamins, and can eventually *cause* constipation.

We offer easy-to-take, inexpensive, nonchemical constipation relievers that should not present any problem side effects if taken in moderation, using good common sense. In other words, don't try more than one remedy at a time.

NOTE: Constipation is a common problem that may be a symptom of disease or lead to more major health problems. It is important to consult with your medical authority before starting any self-help treatment.

‡ CONSTIPATION

The most natural time to move your bowels is within the first few hours of the day. Drinking water on an empty stomach stimulates peristalsis by reflex. So, before breakfast, drink the juice of half a lemon in 1 cup of warm water. While it may help cleanse your system, it may also make you pucker a lot. If you find it hard to drink, sweeten it with honey.

If lemon and water is not for you, eat or drink any one of the following at room temperature (not chilled):

• Prune juice or stewed prunes
• Papaya

- 2 peeled apples
- 6 to 8 dried figs. Soak them overnight in a glass of water. In the morning, drink the water, then eat the figs.

The combination of dried apricots and prunes is said to work wonders. Soak 6 of each overnight. Next morning, eat 3 of each. Then, in the late afternoon, an hour or two before dinner, eat the remaining 3 apricots and 3 prunes.

If you insist on your favorite brand of cereal, add raw, unprocessed bran to it. Start with 1 teaspoon and gradually work your way up to 1 or 2 tablespoons each morning, depending on your reaction to it.

Here are two natural laxatives available at your greengrocer: escarole (eat it raw or boil it in water and drink the water), and Spanish onion (roast it and eat it at bedtime). The cellulose in onions gives intestinal momentum.

Raw sauerkraut and its juice have friendly bacteria and may aid digestion. It's also an excellent laxative. Heat destroys the important enzymes in sauerkraut, so make sure you eat it raw. (Raw sauerkraut is available at health food stores, or see "Preparation Guide" and learn to prepare your own sauerkraut.)

You can also drink the sauerkraut juice to help you overcome constipation. Combine ⅓ of a glass of the juice with ⅔ of a glass of tomato juice and drink it down slowly.

Hippocrates, the father of medicine, recommended eating garlic every day to relieve constipation. Cook with it and eat it raw (in salads) whenever possible.

Just as you're falling asleep, when the mind is most open to autohypnotic suggestion, say to yourself, "In the morning, I will have a good bowel movement." Keep repeating the sentence until you doze off. Pleasant dreams!

‡ MILD LAXATIVES

Raw spinach makes a delicious salad, has lots of vitamins and minerals, and is a mild laxative, too. Be sure to wash it thoroughly.

Aerobic exercise is an excellent laxative.

One teaspoon of blackstrap molasses in ½ cup of warm water an hour before lunch might do the trick.

Soak your feet in cold water, fifteen minutes at a time, once in the morning and once before bedtime. Be sure to dry the feet thoroughly.

Okra acts as a mild laxative. Add chicken gumbo soup to your menu from time to time. Here's a recipe that will give you six delicious servings:

CHICKEN SOUP WITH OKRA
    1 small, cleaned chicken cut into serving portions
    2 tablespoons of flour
    1 onion, chopped
    2 tablespoons of vegetable oil
    4 cups of okra, chopped
    2 cups of tomato pulp
    ¼ cup of parsley, chopped
    4 cups of water
    Salt and pepper
Coat chicken pieces lightly with flour and sauté with onion in oil. Add okra, tomato, parsley, and water as soon as chicken is browned. Season with salt and pepper to taste. Simmer for about two and a half hours, until

chicken is tender and okra is well cooked. Be sure to add water as needed during the two and a half hours of simmering.

‡ STOOL SOFTENER

Every night, before eating dinner, eat a tablespoon of raisins or 3 prunes that have been soaking in water for a couple of hours.

‡Coughs

In the morning, when the doctor examined her patient, she remarked, "I'm happy to say your cough sounds much better."

The patient answered, "Well, it should. I had a whole night of practice."

This may be a joke, but it's not funny if you're the one who's coughing, especially at night, when coughs seem to act up.

We all have a cough center in our brain. It's generally motivated by an irritation in the respiratory tract. In other words, a cough is nature's way of helping us loosen and get rid of mucus that's congesting our system.

Here are some folk remedies that may quell the cough and help you sleep through the night.

NOTE: If cough persists, have it checked by a health professional.

‡ COUGHS IN GENERAL

For five minutes, cook the juice of 1 lemon, 1 cup of honey, and ½ cup olive oil. Then stir vigorously for a couple of minutes.

DOSE: 1 teaspoon every two hours.

Combine ½ cup apple cider vinegar with ½ cup water. Add 1 teaspoon of cayenne pepper and sweeten to taste with honey.

DOSE: 1 tablespoon when the cough starts acting up. Another tablespoon at bedtime.

Peel and finely chop 6 medium onions. Put them and ½ cup of honey into the top of a double boiler, or in a pan over a pot of boiling water. Cover the mixture and let it simmer for two hours. Strain this concoction we call "honion syrup," and pour it into a jar with a cover.

DOSE: 1 warm tablespoon every two to three hours.

Grate 1 teaspoon of horseradish and mix it with 2 teaspoons of honey. (1 finely chopped clove of garlic can be used in place of horseradish.)

DOSE: 1 teaspoon every two to three hours.

For a delicious, thirst-quenching, and soothing drink, squeeze the juice of 1 lemon into a big mug or glass. Add hot water, 2 tablespoons of honey, and either 3 whole cloves, or ½-inch piece of stick cinnamon.

DOSE: One glassful every three hours.

Cook a cup of barley according to the directions on the package. Add the juice of 1 fresh lemon and some water to the cooked barley. Then, liquefy the mixture in a blender. Drink it slowly.

DOSE: One cup every four hours.

Cut a hole through the middle of a rutabaga or a yellow onion and fill the hole with honey or brown sugar. Leave it overnight. In the morning, drink the juice and it will relieve the cough.

Cut a deep hole in the middle of a large beet and fill the hole with honey or brown sugar. Bake the beet until it's soft. It's a treat to eat the beet . . . whenever you feel a cough coming on.

Adding spices and herbs to wine is called mulling. You might want to mull this over for your cough. Into 3 cups of wine, add a 1-inch piece of stick cinnamon, 1 tablespoon of honey, 3 to 6 cloves (depending on how much you like the taste of cloves), and a few pieces of well-scrubbed lemon peel. Heat and stir.

DOSE: 3 cups a day.

Even if this mulled wine doesn't help, you somehow don't mind as much having the cough.

Chew on a bite-size piece of ginger root, just like you would chew gum. Swallowing the juice should help control a cough. Ginger is strong, and it might take some getting used to.

Take a piece of brown grocery-bag paper, about the size of your chest, and soak it in vinegar. When it stops dripping, sprinkle black pepper on one side of the paper. Then place the peppered side on your bare chest. To keep it in place overnight, wrap an Ace bandage or cloth around the chest. By morning, there may be a big improvement, particularly with a bronchial cough.

Among other ingredients, the polyunsaturated fatty acids in whole-grain oats have been said to soothe bronchial inflammation and relieve coughing spasms.

Make a mash from the oats by following the directions on the whole grain oats box, but reduce the amount of water by ¼ cup. Add honey to taste.

DOSE: Eat 1 cup at a time, four times a day and whenever a coughing spell starts. Be sure the oat mash is eaten warm.

‡ DRY COUGH

Take 1 to 2 tablespoons of potato water (see "Preparation Guide") each time the cough acts up. You may want to add honey to taste.

‡ NIGHT COUGH

To help loosen phlegm, fry 2 finely chopped medium onions in lard or vegetable shortening. As soon as it's cool enough to touch, rub the mixture on the cougher's chest and wrap the chest with a clean (preferably white) cloth. Do this procedure in the evening. It may result in a good night's sleep.

Right before bed, add 1 teaspoon of dry mustard powder to a half-filled bathtub of hot water. Prepare a hot drink—take your choice: peppermint tea or hot water, honey, and lemon. Wear bedclothes that leave the chest accessible. Have two rough terrycloth towels and a comfortable chair or stool in the bathroom. Dip your feet in water and keep them there for fifteen minutes. (The rest of the body should be seated alongside the tub.) When the water cools, add more hot water. Sip the drink through this entire process. After fifteen minutes of sipping and dipping (no stripping), dunk the towel in the bathwater, wring it out, and place it on the bare chest. Once the towel cools off, dunk it again, wring it out, and place it back on the chest. Repeat this three times, then dry the body thoroughly, bundle up, and go to bed.

‡ NERVOUS COUGH

We know a stage manager who wants to make this announcement before the curtain goes up: "To stop nervous-type coughs, apply pressure to the area between your lip and your nose. If that doesn't work, press hard on the roof of the mouth. If neither works, please wait till intermission, then go outside and cough."

‡Depression, Stress, and Fatigue

We all go through periods of depression, stress, and fatigue. Maybe it's the weather—you know, a change of season. Or for women, it could be that time of month again. Of course, pressures at the office don't help, nor do tense relationships or problems at home. Then there are additives in foods and side effects from medications that can cause chemical imbalances that can lead to depression, stress, and fatigue.

Whatever the reason, valid or not, when you're going through a bad time and you reach the point where you say to yourself, "I'm sick and tired of being sick and tired!" you're on the road to recovery.

If you are really ready to help yourself, you might start by cutting down on your sugar intake. Excessive sugar can help cause depression, nervous anxiety, and spurts of energy followed by extreme fatigue. Caffeine products (coffee, nonherbal tea, cola, chocolate, and some medications), cigarettes, and alcoholic beverages may also contribute to nervous anxiety, depression, and highs and lows of energy. Take them out of your life. They're taking the life out of you.

Eat a sensible diet of whole grains, steamed green vegetables, lean meat and fish, and raw garlic in big salads with onion and lots of celery. Have sunflower seeds, raisins, sauerkraut, whole wheat pasta, and beans. What could be bad?

For cases of deep depression, extreme stress, and chronic fatigue, we suggest you seek professional assistance to help pinpoint the cause.

Meanwhile, here are some more anxiety-relieving recommendations that may help:

‡ DEPRESSION

Have a pizza with lots of oregano. If you don't have the oregano, forget the pizza. In fact, forget the pizza and just have the oregano. Oregano may ease that depressed, heavy-hearted feeling.

If you have a juicer, whip up half a glass of watercress and half a glass of spinach. Throw in some carrots to make the juice sweeter. Then, bottoms up and spirits up.

Eat 2 ripe bananas a day to chase the blues away. Bananas contain the chemicals serotonin and norepinephrine, which are believed to help prevent depression.

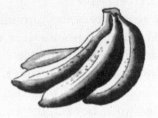

While running a warm bath, prepare a cup of chamomile tea. Add the used tea bag to the bath, along with a new one. If you use loose chamomile, wrap the herb in cheese-cloth before putting it in the tub to avoid messy cleanup. Once the bath is ready, take pen and paper along with your cup of tea and relax in the tub. Make a list of a dozen wishes as you sip your tea. Be careful . . . the things you wish for may come true.

Cheer yourself up by wearing rose colors—pinks and scarlets. The orange family of colors are also picker-uppers.

Making love can help people overcome feelings of depression—unless, of course, they have no one to make love to and that's why they're depressed.

‡ STRESS

Juices seem to be calming to the nerves. Throughout the day, sip apple, pineapple, prune, grape or cherry juice. Make sure the juices have no added sugar or preservatives, and drink them at room temperature, not chilled.

Chop a large onion into very small tidbits and add a tablespoon of honey. Eat half the mixture with lunch and the other half with dinner. Onions contain prostaglandin, which is reported to have a stress-relieving effect.

If strawberries are in season, eat a few as a dessert after each meal (without the cream and sugar!). You may *feel* a difference (you won't be as edgy), and you may *see* a difference (they'll make your teeth whiter).

Acupressure away the pressure of the day by getting a firm grip on your ankle. Using your thumb and third finger, place one just below the inside of the anklebone, and the other finger on the indentation directly below your outer anklebone. Keep steady pressure on the spot as you count down from 100 to 1, slowly (taking between one and two minutes in all).

Peppermint tea has a wonderful way of relaxing the system and relieving moodiness. Drink it warm and strong.

If you are on edge, high-strung, and, generally speaking, a nervous wreck, surround yourself with calming colors. Green has a harmonizing effect, since it's the color of nature. Earth colors should make you feel better. Wear quiet blues and gentle grays. It helps more than we realize.

Sage tea can help relieve the jitters. Steep a sage tea bag or 1 teaspoon of sage in 1 cup of warm water for five minutes. Strain and drink three cups a day. A bonus: Sage tea also helps strengthen one's brain and memory.

There's a reason Epsom salts, an ancient natural healer, is still popular—it works! Pour 2 cups of Epsom salts into a warm-water bath. Set aside one half hour for pure relaxation in the tub—no interruptions—just thirty minutes of stress-free fantasizing.

According to European folklore, celery helps you forget your troubles from a broken heart and soothes your nerves at the same time. It's probably the *phthalide* in celery, which is known to have sedative properties.

‡ NERVOUS TICS

From time to time I get a tic around my eye. I feel like I'm winking at everyone. The tic-off switch that works like magic for me is vitamin B_6—200 mg.

CAUTION: Do not take more than 300 mg of B_6 a day. It can be toxic.

A tic may also be your body's way of telling you that you need more calcium or magnesium or both. A good supplement can help you get the 1,500 mg of calcium and 750 mg of magnesium needed daily.

‡ FATIGUE

If you're tired the second you awaken in the morning, try this Vermont tonic: In a blender, put 1 cup of warm water, 2 tablespoons of apple cider vinegar, and 1 teaspoon of honey. Blend thoroughly, then sip it slowly till it's all gone. Have this tonic every morning before breakfast, and within days, you may feel a difference in your energy level.

A quick picker-upper is ⅛ teaspoon of cayenne pepper in a cup of water. Drink it down and get a second wind.

If you're suffering from mental fatigue, try this Austrian recipe: Thoroughly wash an apple, cut it into small pieces, leaving the peel on, and place the pieces in a bowl. Pour 2 cups of boiling water over the apple and let it steep for an hour. Then add 1 tablespoon of honey. Drink the apple/honey water and eat the pieces of apple.

If possible, walk barefoot in dewy grass. The next best thing is to carefully walk up and back in six inches of cold bathwater. Do it from five to ten minutes in the morning and late afternoon.

If you have a bad case of the drowsies, puncture a garlic pearle (soft gel), or cut a garlic clove in half, and take a few deep whiffs. That ought to wake you up.

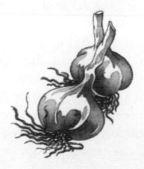

‡Diabetes

In simplified terms, diabetes is a condition in which the pancreas does not produce an adequate amount of insulin to burn up the intake of sugars and starches.

Many cases of diabetes can be completely controlled—controlled, not cured—by a sensible diet. By sticking to a low-calorie, high-carbohydrate diet with plenty of fiber, and exercising (walking at a normal speed for one half hour after every meal), those diabetics remain drug-free and feel better than ever. The importance of controlled weight loss, especially for the obese, cannot be overemphasized.

Thanks to modern laboratory technology, diabetics can perform urinalysis and blood sugar tests conveniently in their own homes. While it makes it easy to monitor oneself, please remember:

DIABETES IS A SERIOUS CONDITION. DO NOT EMBARK ON ANY PLAN OF TREATMENT WITHOUT A DOCTOR'S SUPERVISION.

Along with a well-balanced, sugar-free diet, the combination of garlic, watercress, and parsley, eaten daily, might help regulate the blood sugar level for some diabetics.

Sunchokes, also known as Jerusalem artichokes, although they're not from Jerusalem and they are not artichokes, eaten daily, have been said to help stimulate the production of insulin. They are tubers that contain inulin and levulin, carbohydrates that do not convert to sugar in the body. Jerusalem artichokes are similar in texture to potatoes, but they're sweeter-tasting. They're great for helping you stick to a reducing diet because they satisfy your sweet tooth, and are low in calories and high in vitamins and minerals. Eat them raw as a snack or in salads, boiled in soups, or baked in stews.

Some greengrocers are now carrying them. These tubers are easy to grow and worth the effort if you have the space. Ask your local nursery to help you get started.

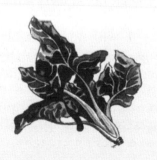

‡Diarrhea and Dysentery

Diarrhea is a common condition usually caused by over-eating, or a minor bacterial infection, or mild food poisoning, and sometimes by emotional anxiety or extreme fatigue.

Even a quick and simple bout of diarrhea depletes the system of potassium, magnesium, and even sodium, often leaving the sufferer tired, depressed, and dehydrated. It's important to keep drinking during and after a siege in order to avoid depletion and dehydration.

NOTE: If diarrhea persists, it may be a symptom of a more serious ailment. Get professional medical attention.

P.S.: "Diarrhea" pronounced backward is "air raid."

‡ DIARRHEA

Since biblical times, the common blackberry plant has been used to cure diarrhea and dysentery. And so the berry remedy, in one form or another, has been passed down through the generations. Don't be surprised if your neighborhood bartender recommends some blackberry brandy.

DOSE: 1 shot glass (2 tablespoons) every four hours.

Blackberry juice or wine will also do fine.

DOSE: 6 ounces blackberry juice every four hours—or 2 ounces (4 tablespoons) blackberry wine every four hours.

Scrape a peeled apple with a (preferably nonmetal) spoon and eat the scrapings. In fact, eat no other food but grated apple until the condition greatly subsides.

Boil ½ cup of white rice in 6 cups of water for one half hour. Strain and save the water, then sweeten with honey to taste.

DOSE: Drink 1 cupful of the rice water every other hour. Do not drink other liquids until the condition disappears.

Eating cooked rice with a dash of cinnamon is also helpful in controlling the problem.

Bananas may help promote the growth of beneficial bacteria in the intestine and replace some of the lost potassium.

DOSE: Three times a day, eat 1 ripe banana that has been soaked in milk.

Add 1 finely chopped teaspoon of garlic to 1 teaspoon of honey and swallow it down three times a day—two hours after each meal.

Lactic acid drinks are effective in treating diarrhea and important in that they replenish the system's supply of friendly intestinal bacteria. Have 1 to 2 glasses of buttermilk or sauerkraut juice or kefir (found in health food stores). Or eat a portion or two of yogurt with active cultures, pickled beets, pickled cucumbers, or raw sauerkraut (see "Preparation Guide" for sauerkraut recipe).

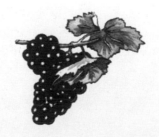

‡ DYSENTERY

It is common for people traveling in foreign countries to get dysentery. All of the above remedies may help treat bacterial dysentery. However, amoebic dysentery (caused by amoeba living in the raw green vegetables of some countries) and viral dysentery are more severe forms of dysentery and should be treated by a health professional. (See "Dysentery" in "And Now May We Prevent . . .")

‡Ears

An earache is generally an infection of the middle ear, usually as a result of a cold or the flu. The pain can be out of proportion to the seriousness of the problem.

In the 1700s, satirist and physicist Georg Lichtenberg said, "What a blessing it would be if we could open and shut our ears as easily as we do our eyes."

If your ears are troubling you, keep your eyes open long enough to read the suggestions that follow.

NOTE: If an earache persists, don't turn a deaf ear! Check it out with a health professional.

IF YOUR EAR IS DRAINING, DO NOT PUT ANYTHING IN IT UNLESS MEDICALLY INSTRUCTED. ONCE YOU'RE SURE THAT THERE IS NO EAR DRAINAGE, CONSIDER USING ANY OF THE FOLLOWING REMEDIES:

‡ EARACHES

Puncture 1 garlic oil soft gel and let the contents ooze into the ear. Gently plug the ear with a puff of cotton. The earache may ease considerably within a half hour.

Combine 4 drops of onion juice (see "Preparation Guide") with 1 teaspoon of warm (not hot), extra virgin, cold-pressed olive oil.

DOSE: 3 drops in each ear in the morning (providing, of course, both ears ache) and 3 drops in each ear in the evening. Be sure to plug the ears with cotton puffs after applying the drops.

Mix ½ cup of unprocessed bran with ½ cup of coarse (kosher) salt and envelop it in a generous piece of folded-over cheesecloth. In other words, bundle it up so it doesn't spill all over the place. Then heat it in a low oven until it's warm but bearable to the touch. Place it on the painful ear and keep it on for an hour.

Put castor oil on a piece of cotton. Sprinkle the oiled cotton with black pepper and apply it to the aching ear— not *in* the ear canal, *on* the ear.

If you're going to get an earache, try to get it when you're baking rye bread. All you have to do is take 1 ounce of caraway seeds and pummel them. Then add 1 cup of bread crumbs from a soft, hot, newly baked loaf of bread and wrap it all in a piece of cheesecloth. Apply it to the sore ear. If you use already-cooled bread, warm the poultice in the oven before applying it.

Most earache remedies say to put something *warm* on the ear. Herbalist Angela Harris feels that the infection-causing bacteria thrive on warmth, and so her approach is with cold on the ear. While an ice pack is on the infected ear, put your feet in hot water—as hot as you can stand it without burning yourself. As if that weren't enough, slowly drink a mild laxative herb tea, available at health food stores. Do this cold, hot, tea remedy for about fifteen minutes, long enough for the pain to be relieved.

‡ INFLAMED EAR

Mix 1 tablespoon of milk with 1 tablespoon of olive oil or castor oil, then heat the combination in a non-aluminum pan.

DOSE: Once the mixture has cooled off, put 4 drops into the inflamed ear every hour and gently plug it up with cotton. Be sure the drops are not too hot.

‡ RUNNY, ABSCESSED EAR

Make a poultice of roasted onion and apply it to the infected ear. It should be as warm as can be without burning that tender, already infected area.

‡ GETTING THE BUGS OUT

It happens! Not often, but once in a blue moon, an insect will get inside a person's ear. Since insects are attracted to light, if an insect gets in your ear, turn toward the sun. Hopefully, the insect will fly out and away. If it occurs at night, shut the lights in the room and shine a flashlight in your ear.

If the insect in your ear doesn't respond to the light, pour 1 teaspoon of warm olive oil into your ear and hold it there a minute or two. Then tilt your head so that the oil and the bug come floating out. If that doesn't work, gently fill your ear with warm water. That should push out the insect and the oil. If none of the above debugs you, get professional medical help to remove the insect.

‡ EAR PAIN IN AIRPLANE

The key to relieving the pressure caused by airplane take-offs and landings is chewing and swallowing.

The American Academy of Otolaryngology advises that

you chew gum or suck on mints—whatever causes you to swallow more than usual. Stay awake as the plane ascends and descends so that you can consciously increase the amount of times you swallow. If you're sleepy, that's good. Hopefully, you'll start yawning, which is even better than swallowing because it activates the muscle that opens your eustachian tube so that air can be forced in and out of your eustachian canal, and that's what relieves the pressure in your ears.

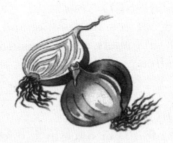

‡ RINGING (TINNITUS)

Ringing in the ears may be the result of a mild overdose of salycilate, which is found in aspirin, or other drugs. The ringing should stop when the drug is discontinued.

If you still hear ringing and there's no one there and you're not in love . . . try onion juice.

DOSE: 2 drops of onion juice in your ears, three times a week should stop the ringing.

Believe it or not, a heating pad on your feet and one on your hands may ease the ringing in your ears. It all has to do with blood being redistributed, improving circulation, and lessening pressure in congested areas.

NOTE: If ringing persists, it might be a sign of a more serious illness, in which case you should seek medical attention.

‡ GETTING THE WAX OUT

Sprinkle black pepper into 1 tablespoon of warm corn oil, then dip a puff of cotton into it and gently put the cotton into your ear. Remove the cotton in five minutes.

Warm 1 tablespoon of 3 percent hydrogen peroxide. Put 10 drops in the ear and let it fizz there for three minutes. Then tilt your head so that the liquid runs out onto a tissue. The wax should be softened. Gently remove the wax with soft cotton. Repeat the procedure with the other ear.

‡ BURNING EARS

Just tell people to stop talking about you!

‡ RESTORE AND/OR IMPROVE HEARING

Pinch the tip of your middle finger four times a day, five minutes each time. It's easy if you organize it this way: before every meal, pinch the right finger. After every meal, pinch the left finger. When you get up in the morning, pinch the right finger. When you go to bed at night, pinch the left finger.

Your right finger is for your right ear and left finger for left ear, so if you want to improve only one ear, pinch accordingly. Make it easy on yourself and clip on a clothespin.

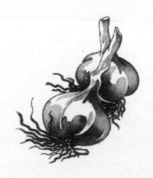

This potent potion has been said to actually restore hearing: drink 1 ounce of garlic juice with 1 ounce of onion juice once a day. [See "Bad Breath" (Halitosis), immediately!]

Nothing improves a person's hearing like overhearing.

NOTE: You should seek professional medical attention for a hearing impairment or sudden hearing loss.

‡ **SWIMMER'S EAR**
Soon after swimming, if you've noticed that it hurts when you touch or move your ear, you may have an ear-canal infection known as "swimmer's ear."
Combine 1 drop of grapefruit extract, 1 drop of tea tree oil, and 2 drops of olive oil and put it in your ear. Gently plug your ear with a cotton puff. This mixture should help clear up the infection.

‡Eyes

How very precious our eyes and sight are to us. Agreed? Agreed! Then what have you done for your eyes lately? Do you know there's eye food, eye-strengthening exercises, an acupressure eyestrain reliever, eyewashes to brighten those baby blues, browns, grays, or greens, and natural healing alternatives instead of chemical symptom cover-ups?

There is an optometrist with a sign in his office window: "If you don't see what you want, you're in the right place."

Likewise. Read the following eye care suggestions, or get someone to read them to you.

‡ STIES

Place a handful of fresh parsley in a soup bowl. Pour a cup of boiling water over the parsley and let it steep for ten minutes. Soak a clean washcloth in the hot parsley water, lie down, put the cloth on your closed lids, and relax for fifteen minutes. Repeat the procedure before bedtime. Parsley water is also good for eliminating puffiness around the eyes.

Moisten a regular (nonherbal) tea bag, put it on the closed eye with the sty, bandage it in place, and leave the bandage on overnight. Hopefully, by morning it will be bye-bye sty.

Rub the sty three times with a gold wedding ring. We decided not to use any silly-sounding, superstition-based remedies. This remedy for sties, however, comes from so many reputable sources that it must have some credibility. Fortunately for us, but unfortunately for research purposes, neither of us has had a sty since working on this book, so we haven't been able to personally test the wedding-ring remedy. In the time you've spent reading all this, you could have rubbed the sty three times and written to tell us if it worked. Could you please do that right now? Thanks. (Our mailing address is in the Introduction.)

‡ CINDERS

If you have something in your eye besides a contact lens, grasp your upper lid lashes firmly between your thumb and index finger. Gently pull the lashes toward the cheek, as far as you can without pulling them out. Hold it, count to 10, spit three times, and let go of the lashes. Is it out? Repeat the procedure one more time. If it still doesn't work, get an onion and read the next remedy.

Mince an onion and let your tears wash away the cinder in your eye.

‡ CHEMICALS

When chemicals like hair dye get in the eye, immediately wash the eye thoroughly with lots of clean, tepid water. In most cases, the eye should be checked by a doctor right after you've washed the damaging liquids out.

‡ CONJUNCTIVITIS (PINKEYE)

Once a day, make a poultice (see "Preparation Guide") of grated apple or grated raw red potato and place it on your closed eye. Let it stay on for one half hour. Within two days, three at the most, the condition should completely clear up.

Prepare chamomile tea. When it cools, use it as an eyewash (see "Preparation Guide") twice a day until the conjunctivitis is gone.

NOTE: Conjunctivitis can be a severe and contagious infection. If the condition doesn't show signs of improvement within a day or two, a health professional should have a look-see.

‡ INFLAMMATIONS AND IRRITATIONS

Peel and slice an overripe apple. Put the pieces of pulp on your closed eyes, holding the pieces in place with a bandage or strip of cloth. Leave it on at least one half hour to help alleviate irritation and inflammation.

A poultice of either grated raw Irish potato, fresh mashed papaya pulp, or mashed cooked beets is soothing and promotes healing. Leave the poultice on for fifteen minutes twice a day.

Reuse used tea bags. Make sure they're moist and cool enough to apply to the closed eyelids for fifteen minutes. This remedy is a favorite for models who wake up puffy-eyed.

‡ BLACK EYES

We met a friend who had a shiner. We asked, "Did someone give you a black eye?" He answered, "No. I had to fight for it."

Eat ripe pineapple and ripe papaya—lots of it—for two or three days, and let the enzymes in those fruits help eliminate the discoloration around the eye. If you can't get fresh pineapple or papaya, try papaya pills (available at health food stores). Take one after every meal. Both fruits are rich in vitamin C, which also promotes healing.

If you were a character in a movie and you got a black eye, in the following scene you would be nursing it with a piece of steak. Cut! The steak may have bacteria that you don't want on your eye, and since the only reason it's being used is because it's cold, retake the scene with a package of frozen vegetables, or a cold wet cloth. Leave it on the bruised area for about twenty minutes, off for ten minutes, on for twenty, off for ten. Get the picture?

Make a poultice by mixing 2 tablespoons of salt with 2 tablespoons of lard or vegetable shortening. Spread the mixture on a cloth and place it over the bruised eye. This poultice may help eliminate the bruised cells around the eye by stimulating the circulation. Be especially careful not to get the salty lard in your eye.

‡ NIGHT BLINDNESS

You know the old joke about carrots being good for your eyes? Well, you've never seen a rabbit wearing glasses. Eat two or three carrots a day (raw or cooked) and/or drink a glass of fresh carrot juice. It's excellent for alleviating night blindness.

Eat blueberries when they're in season. They can help restore night vision.

Eat watercress in salads and/or drink watercress tea.

‡ EYESTRAIN

Pinch the ends of your index and middle (second and third) fingers of each hand. Thirty seconds on each finger.

If your eyestrain isn't relieved after two minutes, do another round of pinching.

Sunflower seeds contain vitamins, iron, and calcium that may be extremely beneficial for eyes. Every day eat about ½ cup of unprocessed (unsalted) shelled seeds.

‡ CATARACTS

There are revolutionary new methods of removing cataracts, where the patient walks in and out of the doctor's office within a few hours. While you're checking into today's modern techniques, you might want to try one or more of the following, to give you some relief until the cataract is professionally removed:

Take 15 mg of vitamin B_2 daily. Also, eat foods high in vitamin B_2: broccoli, salmon, beans, wheat germ, turnip tops, and beets.

Before bedtime, fill an eyedropper with the fresh juice of a coconut and drop in a few drops so that the juice overflows, really washing the eye with the coconut milk. Follow that up with a warm washcloth on the eye for fifteen minutes. (See "Preparation Guide" for instructions on milking a coconut.)

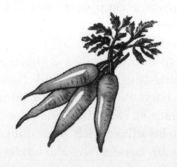

NOTE FOR USING EYEDROPS: To get the most benefit from eyedrops, gently pull out your lower lid and let the liquid drop into the eye pocket. Then keep your eyes closed for about two minutes after putting in the drops. That will prevent the blinking process from pumping the drops out of your eyes.

For five minutes each day, massage the base of the index and middle (second and third) fingers, as well as the webs between those fingers. The right hand helps the right eye and the left hand helps the left eye.

‡ EYE STRENGTHENERS

Apply cold water on a washcloth to the eyelids, eyebrows, and temples, morning, noon, and night, five to ten minutes each time.

Eat about ½ cup of unprocessed (unsalted) sunflower seeds every day.

Put a handful of rose petals (the petals are more potent as the flower fades) into a pot and cover with water. Put it over a medium flame. When the water boils, take the pot off the flame and let it cool. Then strain the water into a bottle and close it tightly. When your eyes feel tired, weak, and red, treat them with the rose petal water. Pour the liquid on a washcloth or cotton pads and keep them on your closed eyes for fifteen to thirty minutes. Your outlook might then be a lot rosier.

This is an interesting way to end the day. Prepare a candle, a straight-back chair, and a five-minute timer. Light the candle and place it one and a half feet from you once you're seated in the chair with your feet uncrossed, flat on the floor. The lit candle should be level with the top of your head. Set the timer for five minutes. Then, using your index fingers, hold your eyelids open while you stare at the candle without blinking. There will be tears. Do not wipe them away. Tough out the five minutes every other night for two weeks. Discontinue the exercise for two weeks. Then start again, every other night for two weeks. Once your vision is sufficiently strengthened, blow out the candle for good.

‡ EYEWASH DIRECTIONS

Reminder: *Always remove contact lenses before doing an eyewash.*

You'll need an eye cup (available at drugstores). Carefully pour just-boiled water over the cup to clean it. Without contaminating the rim or inside surfaces of the cup, fill it half full with whichever eyewash you've selected. Apply the cup tightly to the eye to prevent spillage, then tilt your head backward. Open your eyelid wide and rotate your eyeball to thoroughly wash the eye. Use the same procedure with the other eye.

‡ EYEWASH FOR BRIGHT, CLEAR EYES

Place a handful of scrubbed carrot tops in a jar of distilled hot water. Let it stand. When it's cool, use the carrot water as an eyewash. Drink the remaining liquid. It should help your eyes and also help strengthen your kidneys and bladder.

Mix 1 drop of lemon juice in 1 ounce of distilled warm water and use it as an eyewash. It's particularly effective when your eyes have been exposed to dust, cigarette smoke, harsh lights, and chemical compounds in the air.

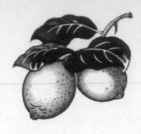

‡ SUNBURNED EYES
See "Burns."

‡Feet and Legs

"Oh, my aching feet!" is a common cry heard 'round the world.

Our feet carry a lot of weight and are probably the most abused and neglected part of our anatomy. At some time or other, we're all guilty of the Cinderella Stepsister syndrome—pushing our feet into ill-fitting shoes.

We put our poor, tired tootsies under all kinds of stress and strain. They get cold, they get frostbitten, they get wet, they burn, they blister, they itch, they sweat, as we walk, jog, run, dance, climb, skate, ski, hop, skip, and jump. Then we wonder why our feet are "just killing us!" Well, we killed them first.

Let's get to the bottom of our troubles with some remedies for the feet.

‡ CORNS

The difference between an oak tree and a tight shoe is that one makes acorns, the other makes corns ache. Now, what to do for those aching corns:

Rub castor oil on the corn twice a day and it will gradually peel off, leaving soft, smooth skin.

Every night, put 1 piece of fresh lemon peel on the corn (the inside of the peel on the outside of the corn). Put a

Band-Aid around it to keep it in place. In a few days, the corn should be gone.

Make a poultice of 1 crumbled piece of bread soaked in ¼ cup of vinegar. Let it stand for half an hour, then apply it to the corn and tape it in place overnight. By morning, the corn should peel off. If it's a particularly stubborn corn, you may have to reapply the bread/vinegar poultice a few nights in a row.

Every day, wrap a strip of fresh pineapple peel around the corn (the inside of the peel taped directly on the corn). Within a week, the corn should disappear, thanks to the enzymes and acid content of the fresh pineapple.

Hell hath no fury like a woman's corn! Here are another couple of remedies:

Don't throw away used tea bags. Tape a moist one on the corn for one half hour a day and the corn should be gone in a week or two.

To ease the pain of a corn, soak the feet in oatmeal water. Bring 5 quarts (20 cups) of water to a boil and add 5 ounces (1⅔ cups) of oatmeal. Keep boiling until the water boils down to about 4 quarts. Then pour off the clear water through a strainer, into a large enough basin for your feet, or into two plastic shoe boxes. Soak your feet for at least twenty minutes.

‡ ATHLETE'S FOOT

The fungus that causes athlete's foot dies in natural sunlight. So, if you can spend the next two weeks barefoot in the Bahamas . . . If that's a bit impractical, then for one hour a day, expose your feet to sunlight and that might eliminate a mild case of athlete's foot.

In between sunbaths, keep the feet well aired by wearing loose-fitting socks. At night, apply alcohol (Ow! it stings for a couple of seconds), then wait till your feet are very dry and sprinkle on talcum powder (the unscented kind is preferable).

Apply 1 clove of crushed garlic to the affected area. Leave it on for half an hour, then wash with water. If you do this once a day, within a week, you'll be smelling like a salami, but you may not have athlete's foot.

CAUTION: When you first apply the garlic, there will be a sensation of warmth for a few minutes. If, after a few minutes, that warm feeling intensifies and the garlic is burning the skin, wash the area with cool water. The next day, dilute garlic juice with water and try again.

Every evening, apply cotton or cheesecloth that has been saturated with honey to the infected area. Tape it in place. To avoid a gooey mess (a possibility even with the tape in place), wear socks to bed. In the morning, wash with water, dry thoroughly, and sprinkle on (preferably unscented) talcum powder. In a week's time, you may have every bear in the neighborhood at your feet, but they probably won't be athlete's-foot feet.

To avoid reinfecting yourself with athlete's foot, soak your socks and hose in vinegar. Also wipe out your shoes with vinegar.

‡ ACHING FEET
During a busy day when your "dogs are barking" and you feel like you're going to have to call it quits, cayenne pepper to the rescue! Sprinkle some cayenne into your socks, or rub it directly on the soles of your aching feet. Now get going or you'll be late for your next appointment!

After a long day, when your nerves are on edge, your feet hurt, you're tired—too tired to go to sleep—soak your feet in hot water for ten to fifteen minutes. Then (this is the important part) massage your feet with lemon juice. After you've done a thorough job of massaging, rinse your feet with cool water. As always, dry your feet completely, then take five deep breaths. You and your pain-free feet should be ready and able to settle down for a good night's sleep.

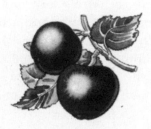

‡ BURNING FEET
Wrap tomato slices on the soles of the feet and keep the feet elevated for half an hour.

Soak your feet in warm potato water (see "Preparation Guide") for fifteen minutes. Dry your feet thoroughly. If you're going right to bed, massage the feet with a small amount of sesame or almond oil. You might want to put on loose-fitting socks to avoid messing up the sheets.

Bavarian mountain climbers, after soaking their feet in potato water, sprinkle hot, roasted salt on a cloth and wrap it around their feet. It not only soothes burning and tired feet, but relieves itchy ones as well.

‡ COLD FEET
Stand on your toes for a couple of minutes, then quickly come back down on your heels. Repeat toes/heels several

times until your blood tingles through your feet and warms them up.

Before going to bed, walk in cold water in the bathtub for two minutes. Then briskly rub the feet dry with a coarse towel. To give the feet a warm glow, hold each end of the towel and run it back and forth through the hollow of the feet.

If the thought of putting already cold feet into cold water is not appealing to you, then add 1 cup of table salt to a bathtub filled, ankle-high, with hot water and soak the feet for fifteen minutes. Dry the feet and massage them with damp salt. This will remove dead skin and stimulate circulation. After you've rubbed each foot for three to five minutes, rinse them both in lukewarm water and dry them thoroughly.

Warm your feet by sprinkling black pepper or cayenne pepper into your socks before putting them on. It's an old skier's trick, but you don't have to be an old skier to do it. If you use cayenne, your socks and your feet will turn red. Your feet will be fine, but your socks may never be the same again.

Oh, and if you're at a restaurant and the food is too bland, you can always take off a sock and season to taste.

‡ PIGEON-TOES

If you are slightly pigeon-toed and an orthopedist hasn't helped you, as a last resort, buy a pair of shoes one size larger than you usually take. Wear them to bed every night with the right shoe on the left foot and the left shoe on the right foot. Give it a month to get results.

‡ LEG CRAMPS

Drink a glass of tonic water. It may have enough quinine to help you and not enough to harm you.

If you get leg cramps while you sleep, keep a piece of silverware—a spoon seems the safest—on your night table. When the cramp wakes you up, place the spoon on the painful area and the muscle should uncramp. Incidentally, the spoon doesn't have to be silver; stainless steel will work as well.

Cramp bark is an herb that—you guessed it—is good for any sort of cramping. The tincture is available at health food stores. Take 1 to 2 teaspoons three to five times a day.

‡Female Problems

We've come a long way, baby!

Today, we talk openly about menstruation, pregnancy, and menopause, not as sicknesses, but as natural stages of life. We also recognize and deal with premenstrual tension, menstrual pain, and menopausal irregularities.

And we are finally learning to question the male-dominated medical profession after hearing countless stories about hysterectomies, radical mastectomies, and other surgery that's sometimes performed whether a woman needs it or not.

Remember, knowledge is power. Television talk shows, the Internet, bookstores, and local libraries are filled with women's health information. Take advantage of these sources so that you can intelligently and happily take responsibility for your own body, your choices for professional medical care, and for good health.

Meanwhile, here are some home remedies whispered down from generation to generation.

‡ BRINGING ON MENSTRUATION

NOTE: NONE OF THESE REMEDIES WILL WORK IF YOU ARE PREGNANT OR DO NOT HAVE A UTERUS.

To help bring on and regulate menstruation, eat and drink fresh beets and beet juice. Have about 3 cups of beets and juice each day past your due-date until the flow begins.

A footbath in hot water has been said to help bring on a delayed menstrual period.

Add 1 tablespoon of basil to a cup of boiling water. Let it steep for five minutes. Strain and drink.

In a circular motion, massage below the outer and inner ankle of each foot, as well as the outer and inner wrist of each hand. If there is tenderness when you rub those areas, you're in the right place. Keep massaging until the tenderness is gone. Chances are your problem will also soon be gone. Within a day or two, your period should start.

Ginger tea can stimulate the onset of menstruation. Put four or five quarter-size pieces of fresh ginger in a cup of just-boiled water and let it steep for ten minutes. Drink 3 or 4 cups of the tea throughout the day. It also helps ease menstrual cramps.

‡ EXCESSIVE MENSTRUAL FLOW

NOTE: Hemorrhaging requires immediate medical attention! If you are not sure about the difference between hemorrhaging and excessive menstrual flow, do not take a chance—if you are bleeding profusely, get medical attention quickly. If your menstrual flow is excessive, the following remedies have been said to help. We also suggest you have a checkup.

Mix the juice of ½ lemon into a cup of warm water. Drink it down slowly an hour before breakfast and an hour before dinner.

Throughout the day, sip cinnamon tea made with a piece of cinnamon stick steeped in hot water. Or use 4 drops of cinnamon bark tincture in a cup of warm water.

When bleeding excessively, stay away from alcoholic beverages and hot, spicy foods, except for cayenne pepper. (See next remedy.)

Add ⅛ of a teaspoon of cayenne pepper to a cup of warm water or your favorite herbal tea and drink it. Cayenne pepper is a powerful bleeding regulator.

To help control profuse menstrual flow, it's time for thyme tea. Steep 2 tablespoons of thyme in 2 cups of hot water. Let it stand for ten minutes. Strain and drink 1 cup. Add an ice cube to the other cup of tea, then soak a washcloth in it and use it as a cold compress on the pelvic area.

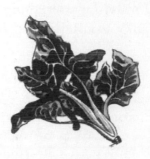

‡ PREMENSTRUAL TENSION AND PERIOD PAINS

Chamomile tea is a superb tension reliever and nerve relaxer. As soon as menstrual cramps start, prepare chamomile tea and sip it throughout the day.

Premenstrual tension as well as menstrual cramps may be relieved by increasing calcium intake. Menopausal symptoms may also be prevented by adding calcium to the diet. On a daily basis, it is a good idea to eat at least one portion of two or three of these calcium-rich foods: leafy green vegetables (collard greens, dandelion greens, kale, mustard greens, broccoli, turnip greens, watercress, parsley, endive), canned salmon, sardines and anchovies, figs, and yogurt.

Minimize or completely eliminate caffeine and alcoholic beverages. They increase the amount of calcium lost in the urine.

Check with a health professional before taking a calcium supplement. They've been known to cause kidney stones in some people.

Peppermint tea is soothing. It also helps digestion and rids you of that bloated feeling. Drink a cup of peppermint tea after (not during) your meal.

For premenstrual relief for everything from the blues to breast tenderness, take two garlic supplements daily.

‡ MENOPAUSE

A Viennese gynecologist has reported positive results among his female patients treated with bee pollen. Bee pollen contains a combination of male and female hormones. It has been known to help some women do away with or minimize the hot flashes.

DOSE: 3 bee pollen pills (500 mg) a day, or the granule equivalent.

The estrogenic substances in black cohosh may relieve menopause symptoms, like hot flashes and even vaginal dryness. You'll find the herb in tincture form at health food stores. Follow the recommended dosage on the label.

If you have excessive menstrual flow during menopause, mix 1 ounce of grated nutmeg in 1 pint of Jamaican rum.

DOSE: Take 1 teaspoon three times a day for the duration of your period.

Eat a cucumber every day. Cukes are said to contain beneficial hormones.

‡ MASTITIS

Mastitis is an inflammation of the breast. The two common kinds are acute mastitis, involving bacterial infection, and chronic mastitis, often with no infection—just tenderness and pain.

This condition should be checked out by a health professional.

If you have a bacterial infection, chances are you will be treated with antibiotics. Antibiotics have no discretion. They destroy the good as well as the bad bacteria. Replace the beneficial bacteria with Lactobacillus acidophilus. You can do that by eating yogurt—make sure the container says *Live* or *Active Culture with L. acidophilus*—or by taking an acidophilus supplement, available at health food stores. Whether you take an acidophilus supplement or eat yogurt (fat-free is fine as long as it says it contains *L. acidophilus*), take it two hours after taking an antibiotic. Allow that amount of time so that it doesn't interfere with the work of the antibiotic. Keep consuming acidophilus in some form for at least a couple of weeks after you stop taking the antibiotics. It will help normalize the bacterial balance in the intestines, getting your digestive system working properly again.

To relieve the tenderness and pain of mastitis, place a cabbage leaf on your breast, and let your bra hold it in place. According to herbalist Angela Harris, the cabbage draws out the toxins and the pain.

‡ CYSTITIS

Pour a small box of baking soda into a bath of warm water and soak in it for at least a half hour, then rinse under the shower.

Even some physicians now prescribe cranberry juice for cystitis. You can get juice that's sugarless with no added preservatives at most supermarkets, or you can buy cranberry concentrate (which needs to be diluted) at health food stores, or use cranberry capsules and follow the dosage on the label.

JUICE DOSE: One 8-ounce glass in the morning, before breakfast, and one glass in the late afternoon. Make sure it's at room temperature, not chilled.

Take 2 garlic capsules a day and, if you don't mind smelling like a salami, drink garlic tea throughout the day. Mash a couple of garlic cloves into hot water and let them steep for five minutes. You can also make garlic tea with 1 teaspoon of garlic powder in hot water.

NOTE: Persistent cystitis may require antibiotics prescribed by a doctor. If that is the case, be sure to eat yogurt with live or active cultures, during and after taking the antibiotics.

‡ FEMALE PROBLEMS IN GENERAL

Gently but firmly, massage the back of the leg, around the ankle. Massaging that area can relax tension, stimulate circulation, and soothe the female organs.

‡ VAGINITIS (INFECTIONS)

Wear cotton panties to absorb moisture, since moisture encourages the growth of organisms. For that reason, stay away from moisture-inducing garments like panty hose, girdles, leotards, tights, Spandex, etc.

Take showers instead of baths. Baths can add to your problems when the vaginal area is exposed to bathwater impurities.

Do not use any chemical products such as feminine hygiene sprays. Also, avoid tampons and colored or scented toilet tissue.

Do not launder panties along with socks, stockings, or other undergarments. Wash panties separately with a mild soap or detergent and rinse them very thoroughly.

Place a poultice of cottage cheese, or farmer cheese, or yogurt with active cultures on a sanitary napkin and wear it. Change the poultice every three to five hours. Hopefully, the itching will stop rather quickly and the infection will be gone within a week or two.

‡ FRIGIDITY

Frigidity often stems from a lack of communication between a woman and her man. Sex counseling may be the necessary remedy.

As for the "Not tonight, honey" syndrome, eating a piece of halvah may awaken sexual desires. This Middle Eastern treat is made of sesame seeds and honey. The sesame seeds are high in magnesium and potassium. Honey has aspartic acid. All three substances have been said to help women overcome lack of lust.

Licorice has female hormones in it. In France it might not be uncommon to see women drink licorice water, believing it may improve their love life. Powdered licorice is available at health food stores. Drink 1 teaspoon in a cup of water and get out the black lingerie. If you have high blood pressure, use the lingerie, but *NOT* the licorice.

‡ PREGNANCY: DURING AND AFTER

Morning Sickness

If you are troubled by morning sickness, check with your obstetrician about taking 50 mg of vitamin B_6 and 50 mg of vitamin B_1 daily. Since garlic greatly increases the body's absorption of B_1, make an effort to eat garlic raw in salads and to cook with it.

Constipation During Pregnancy

Keep a chair, stool, or carton in the bathroom so that you can rest your feet on it when you're on the toilet seat. Once your feet are on the same level as the seat, lean back and relax. To avoid hemorrhoids and varicose veins, do not strain and do not hold your breath and squeeze.

Increase Mother's Milk After Pregnancy

Bring to a boil 1 teaspoon of caraway seeds in 8 ounces of water. Then, simmer for five minutes. Let it cool and drink. Several cups of caraway seed tea a day may increase mother's milk supply.

Brewer's yeast (available at health food stores) may also help.

‡ CRACKED AND/OR SORE NIPPLES

When herbalist Angela Harris was nursing any one of her eight children, between nursings, she would moisten a black tea bag (usually Lipton's Orange Pekoe) and apply it to her cracked or sore nipple. It relieved the pain and helped heal the cracking.

‡Frostbite

The extent of frostbite varies greatly, depending on the length of time a person has been exposed to the cold; the intensity of the cold, humidity, winds; the kinds and amount of clothing worn; a person's natural resistance to cold, as well as a person's general health.

One big problem with frostbite is that it's hard to know you have it until it's on its way to being serious.

At some ski resorts, the ski patrol does occasional nose and cheek checks of skiers. Thanks to those checks, lots of mild frostbite victims are sent indoors to defrost.

Seriously frostbitten victims should be placed under a doctor's care and/or hospitalized immediately.

Be sure the frostbite sufferer is in a warm room while waiting for medical help. If the person is conscious, give him or her a warm drink. NO ALCOHOLIC BEVERAGES! They can worsen the condition. The frozen body parts must be warmed slowly. Be careful when touching the skin not to break the frostbite blisters. Cover the frostbitten areas with a blanket or warm (not hot) water. If it's warm, running water, make sure it runs gently over the skin.

For mild cases of frostbite, all of the above apply; in addition, the following remedies are worth a try.

Steep a teaspoon of sage in a cup of hot water for five minutes and drink it. Sage tea will help improve circulation.

When we were kids, we saw a cartoon of a male Eskimo urinating ice cubes. Funny? Yes. Accurate? No. No matter how cold we are, our urine stays fairly warm. If you're indoors and without warm water, apply your own urine to your frostbitten areas. It should help you thaw out.

Pour witch hazel over the frostbitten areas.

Warm some olive oil and gently dab it on the frostbitten skin or paint it on with a kitchen pastry brush.

If you have an aloe vera plant or bottled aloe vera gel, gently apply it to the area.

Boil and mash potatoes. Add salt and apply the mixture to the frostbitten areas. If you're hungry, eat the potatoes and apply the warm water in which the potatoes were boiled to the frostbitten areas.

‡Hair

According to a French proverb, "A fool's hair never turns white." The Russians say, "There was never a saint with red hair." "Pull out a gray hair," according to the German Pennsylvanians, "and seven will come to its funeral."

Hair is a secondary sex characteristic and seems to, appropriately, play a part in sexual attractiveness.

The biggest hair worries: too much or too little. Too much hair, especially in the wrong places, can be permanently removed by electrolysis. It's expensive and painful, but worth every penny and pain in exchange for a better self-image.

Too little hair, especially in men, is usually hereditary baldness (alopecia). If none of the available hair-restoring treatments including cosmetic surgery (implants and transplants) and the drugs currently on the market are for you, you may want to try one of the folk remedies that people claim have stopped the loss of hair as well as restored the hair already lost. Neither of us has seen it happen to anyone we know. It may be worth a try. After all, what do you have to lose that you aren't already losing?

‡ STOPPING LOSS AND PROMOTING GROWTH

An hour before bedtime, slice open a clove of garlic and rub it on the hairless area. An hour later, massage the scalp with olive oil, put on a slumber cap, and go to bed. The next morning, shampoo. Repeat the procedure night and morning for a few weeks and, hopefully, hair will have stopped falling out and there will be regrowth showing.

Three times a day, five minutes each time, buff your fingernails with your fingernails. Huh? In other words, rub the fingernails of your right hand across the fingernails of your left hand. Not only is it supposed to stop hair loss, it's also supposed to encourage hair growth and prevent hair from graying.

Prepare your own hair-growing elixir by combining ¼ cup of onion juice with 1 tablespoon of honey. Massage the scalp with the mixture every day. We heard about a man who had a bottle of this hair tonic. One day, he took the cork out of the bottle with his teeth. The next day, he had a mustache that needed to be trimmed. But seriously . . .

DO NOT DO THIS EXERCISE IF YOU HAVE HIGH OR LOW BLOOD PRESSURE! DO NOT DO THIS EXERCISE WITHOUT YOUR DOCTOR'S APPROVAL IF YOU ARE SIGNIFICANTLY BEYOND YOUNG ADULTHOOD! Stand on your head. If you can't, then get down on all fours, with your hands about two feet from your knees. Then carefully lift your rear end in the air so that your legs are straight and your head is between your outstretched arms. Stay in that position for a minute each day, and after a week, gradually work your way up to five minutes each day. The theory behind this is that you will bring oxygen to the hair bulbs, which will rejuvenate the scalp and encourage hair to grow.

‡ DRY HAIR
Shampoo and towel-dry your hair. Then, evenly distribute 1 tablespoon of mayonnaise throughout your hair. (Use more if your hair is long.) After the mayonnaise has been

on for an hour, wash hair with a mild shampoo and rinse. The theory is that the flow of oil from the sebaceous glands is encouraged as the natural fatty acids of the mayonnaise help nourish the hair.

‡ FRIZZY DRY HAIR

After shampooing, rinse with 1 tablespoon of wheat germ oil, followed by a mixture of ½ cup of apple cider vinegar and 2 cups of water. It will tame the frizzies.

‡ HAIR REVITALIZER

This was our mom's favorite hair treatment. (Actually, it was the only hair treatment she ever used.) Slightly warm ½ cup of olive oil. You may want to add a few drops of an extract like vanilla, to make it more fragrant. Mom put it in an eyedropper bottle and let it stand in very hot water for a few minutes. Then, using the eyedropper, she'd put the warm oil on the hair and massage it into the scalp. Once the whole head is oiled, shampoo the oil out.

‡ DULL PERMED HAIR

After shampooing, rinse with a combination of 1 cup of apple cider vinegar and 2 cups of water. Your hair will come alive and shine. This treatment is especially effective on permed hair, but can be used on any lifeless-looking hair.

‡ THIN, BODILESS HAIR

Add 2 egg whites and the juice of ½ lemon to your shampoo. This will give your hair more body and volume.

‡ DANDRUFF

Wash your hair with a combination of 1 cup of beet juice and 2 cups of water, plus 1 teaspoon of salt. This is an Arabian remedy. Remember, Arabs have dark hair. Since beets contain a dye, this is not recommended for light-haired people who want to stay that way. To be safe, do a test on a patch of hair.

Squeeze the juice of 1 large lemon and apply half of it to your hair. Mix the other half with 2 cups of water. Wash your hair with a mild shampoo, then rinse with water. Rinse again with the lemon and water mixture. Repeat every other day until dandruff disappears.

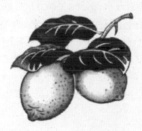

‡ MAKING GREEN HAIR DISAPPEAR

Don't you just hate it when you get out of the pool and your blonde hair has a greenish tinge? Next time, take a clean sponge, dip it in red wine, and dab it on your 'do. The chemicals in a chlorinated pool will be neutralized by the tannic acid in the wine.

Keep a bottle of lemon juice and a box of baking soda in your locker. After your swim, and before you hit the shower, mix ½ cup of the baking soda into a cup of lemon juice. Wet your hair, then rinse it with this bubbly mixture to get the green out. (Maybe blondes *don't* have more fun.)

‡ A RINSE FOR SHINIER DARK HAIR

Prepare a rinse in a glass or ceramic bowl. Add 3 tablespoons of either parsley or rosemary or sage (available at herb and health food stores) to 8 cups of just-boiled water. Let it steep until it gets cool. Strain through muslin, or a superfine strainer. After shampooing, massage the herb water into your scalp as you rinse with it.

‡ A RINSE FOR SHINIER FAIR HAIR

Prepare a rinse in a glass or ceramic bowl. Add 3 tablespoons of either chamomile or calendula or yarrow (available at herb and health food stores) to 8 cups of just-boiled water. Let it steep until it gets cool. Strain through muslin, or a superfine strainer. After shampooing, massage the herb water into your scalp as you rinse with it.

‡Headaches

Take a holistic approach to yourself and your headache. Step back and look at the past twenty-four hours of your life. Have you eaten sensibly? Did you get a decent night's sleep? Have you moved your bowels since awakening this morning? Are there deadlines you need to meet? Do you have added pressures at home or at work? Is there something you're dreading?

Now that you probably realize the reason for your headache, what should you take for it? Don't refuse any offer.

Since studies show that more than 90 percent of headaches are brought on by nervous tension, most of our remedies are for the common tension headache and a few for the more serious migraines.

In the case of regularly recurring headaches, they can be caused by eyestrain, an allergy, or something more serious. We suggest you seek professional medical attention.

Headaches are a headache! Use your instincts, common sense, and patience to find what works best for you and your headache.

‡ HEADACHES IN GENERAL

When our grandmother had a headache, she would dip a large white handkerchief in vinegar, wring it out, and tie it tightly around her forehead until the headache disappeared.

A variation of soaking a handkerchief in vinegar is to soak a piece of brown grocery-bag paper in vinegar. Shake off the excess liquid and place it on your forehead. Tie it in place and keep it there for at least one half hour.

Peel the rind off a lemon. Make the pieces as wide as possible. Rub the rind (the inside of the skin should touch your skin) on your forehead and temples. Then place the rind on the forehead and temples, securing them with a scarf or bandage. Keep it there until the headache goes away, usually within a half hour.

Let ice-cold water accumulate, ankle-high, in the bathtub. Dress warmly except for your bare feet. Take a leisurely stroll in the tub—from one to three minutes—as long as it takes for your feet to start feeling warm in the ice-cold water. When that happens, get out of the tub, dry your feet, and go directly to bed. Cover up, relax, and within no time, your headache should be a pain of the past.

Press your thumb against the roof of your mouth for four to five minutes. Every so often, move your thumb to another section of the roof of your mouth. The nerve pressure in your head should be greatly relieved. While it's highly impractical during a speaking engagement, it's worth a try in the privacy of your home.

Mix a cup of water with a cup of apple cider vinegar and bring it to a slow boil in a medium-size pot. When the fumes begin to rise, reduce the flame as low as it will get. Put a towel over your head, bend over the pot (be careful: steam can burn if you get too close), and inhale and exhale deeply through your nose about eighty times or for about ten minutes. Be sure to hold the towel so that it doesn't catch fire, but catches the vapor for you to inhale.

If strawberries are in season, eat a few. They contain organic salicylates, which are like the active ingredients in aspirin.

Vigorously rub the second joint of each thumb, two minutes on the right hand, two minutes on the left hand, until you've done it five times each, or for ten minutes. Use hand lotion on the thumbs to eliminate friction.

A very old American remedy to swallow is a teaspoon of honey mixed with ½ teaspoon of garlic juice.

During my est training, I was told that whatever you fully experience, disappears. This est process can help you experience away your headache. Ask yourself the following questions and answer them honestly:

- Do you *really* want to get rid of the headache? (Don't laugh. A lot of people want to hang on to their headaches. It's a great excuse and cop-out from all kinds of things.)
- What kind of headache is it? Be specific. Is it a pounding over one eye? Does it throb each time you bend down? Do you have a dull ache at the base of your neck? Now, either learn the next questions by heart or have someone read them to you. ("Why?" you wonder.) Close your eyes. ("Aha!" That's why.)
- What size is your headache? Describe the exact dimensions of it. Start with the length from the front of your face to the back of your head, the width from ear to ear and the thickness of it from the top of your head down toward your neck.
- What color is your headache?
- How much water will it hold? (This is done in your mind through visualization.) Fill a cup with the amount of water needed to fill the area of the headache. Then, pour the water from the cup into the space of your headache. When you've completed that, open your eyes. You should have experienced away your headache. The first time I used this process, my results were quite

dramatic. If I hadn't experienced it myself, I'd probably think it's as crazy as you're probably thinking I am right now.

Enlist the help of someone who will slowly move his or her thumb down the right side of your back, alongside your shoulder blade and toward your waist. Let that person know when (s)he hits a sore or tender spot. Have your helpmate exert steady pressure on that spot for a minute. By then you should have relief from the headache.

‡ SINUS HEADACHES
Sniff a little horseradish juice—the stronger the horseradish, the better. Remember to do it slowly.

Prepare poultices of either raw grated onion or horseradish. Apply the poultices to the nape of the neck and the soles of the feet. Leave them on for an hour.

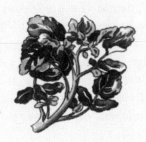

‡ MIGRAINES
Dip a few cabbage leaves in boiling hot water to make them soft. As soon as they're cool enough, place one or two thicknesses on your forehead and on the back of your neck. Secure them in place with a scarf or bandage. Then relax as the cabbage draws out the pain.

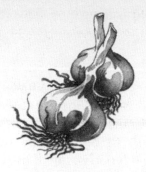

Boil 2 Spanish onions. Eat one and mash the other for a poultice. Then place the poultice on your forehead.

Apply pressure to the palm of one hand with the thumb of the other hand. Then, reverse the order. If you feel a tenderness in either palm, concentrate the massage on that area. Keep up the firm pressure and massage for ten minutes—five minutes on each hand.

We heard about a woman who would take a tablespoon of honey the second she felt a migraine coming on. If the headache wasn't gone within a half hour, she'd take another tablespoon of honey with three glasses of water and that would do it.

NOTE: Chronic migraine sufferers should seek medical attention.

‡Heart

The heart is a four-chambered hollow muscle and double-acting pump located in the chest between the lungs. This hardworking, fist-size muscle pumps blood through the blood vessels in all parts of the body at the rate of about 4,000 gallons a day. (No wonder so many of us have "tired blood.")

The heart is so complex and heart trouble is so serious that the best suggestions we can offer are:

- If you feel as though you're having a heart attack, call for professional medical help IMMEDIATELY!
- If you have a history of heart problems, follow an eating plan that will promote a healthy heart. (See our "Suggested Reading" list.)
- To help others, take a cardiac pulmonary resuscitation (CPR) course through your local Red Cross chapter.
- Don't smoke!

‡ HEART STRENGTHENERS

While doing research, we found some things that may help strengthen the heart. We'd like to share them with you, with the understanding that these *do not* take the place of professional medical attention.

Omega-3 oils impact many factors linked to cardiovascular disease. They help lower LDL-cholesterol levels and triglycerides, inhibit excessive platelet aggregation, lower fibrinogen levels, and lower both systolic and diastolic blood pressure in individuals with high blood pressure. Flaxseed oil offers the most cost effective and beneficial method for increasing the intake of omega-3 oils in the diet. (See "And Now May We Prevent . . ." for detailed *flaxseed oil* information.)

For a healthier heart, eat wheat germ every day. You might want to supplement the wheat germ with vitamin E (400 I.U.). It's said to help reduce hardening of the arteries.

If you have palpitations occasionally, as most of us do, drink peppermint tea. Have a mugful a day. It seems to have a calming effect on people, especially since it is an herb tea that does not have caffeine.

Beware that peppermint is a powerful herb that can undermine or negate the effectiveness of homeopathic medicine.

Take a garlic supplement every day to protect and strengthen the heart and help thin the blood. Also, use garlic in cooking and raw in salads.

Moderate consumption of red wine, as reported in England's respected medical journal *The Lancet,* is directly associated with lower rates of heart disease.

According to wine therapists, a little champagne sipped daily helps strengthen the heart. The champagne's tartrate of potassium content supposedly has a positive effect on one's cardiac rhythm.

(Please remember, EVERYTHING IN MODERATION!)

We've been told that massaging the pads at the base of the last two fingers of the left hand, or massaging the left foot under the third, fourth, and fifth toes, can relieve heart pain within seconds.

If someone wants to give you an edible treat, instead of candy suggest red roses. They're said to help strengthen the heart as well as other organs of the body, not to mention what they do for a relationship. Remove the bitter white part on the bottom of the petals and eat the rest of the petals raw, or make rose petal tea to drink. Be sure the roses are organically grown and haven't been sprayed. There are tribes in India who live on roses alone. They don't have their groceries delivered. They send flowers by wire.

Eat onions once a day. According to Russian scientists, onions are good for all kinds of heart problems.

Every morning, before breakfast, drink the juice of half a lemon in a cup of warm water. It's reputed to be helpful for all kinds of body functions from proper fluid action in the blood to regularity in the bathroom.

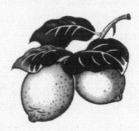

‡ CHOLESTEROL

The only foods that have cholesterol are animal products—meat, poultry, fish, dairy. If you have high cholesterol, start a heart-smart diet immediately by cutting down or cutting out animal products. There are foods that can help lower your LDL (bad cholesterol) and raise your HDL (good cholesterol).

There have been a variety of cholesterol studies conducted over different periods of time with any number of test subjects. Some of the results are impressive, and all of the cholesterol-lowering foods are worth a try. First, and most important, is to get that heart-smart diet in place, and incorporate the foods listed below.

- Eating two large apples a day caused cholesterol levels to drop 16 percent. That may be because apples are rich in flavonoids and pectin. Pectin may form a gel in the stomach that keeps fats in food from being totally absorbed.

- Eating ½ avocado a day may lower cholesterol by 8 to 42 percent. Yes, they're high in fat, but it's mono-unsaturated fat that does good things for the system. Avocado also contains thirteen essential minerals, including iron, copper, and magnesium, and is rich in potassium. It tastes great, too.

- Eating 2 raw carrots a day reduced cholesterol levels by 11 percent.

- People who consumed about ¾ cup of fenugreek daily for twenty days cut their LDL (bad cholesterol) levels by 33 percent; their HDL (good cholesterol) happily stayed the same. Instead of having to eat tablespoons of ground fenugreek seeds, choose capsules (580 mg), available at health food stores. Take one or two with each meal.

- Eating about 4 cloves of garlic a day can cut total cholesterol by about 7 percent. (While fresh garlic is best, garlic supplements are next best.)

- Taking 1,000 mg of vitamin C a day for eight months, men and women who started out with low blood levels of vitamin C had a 7 percent increase of their HDL (good cholesterol) readings.

- Kiwi has what it takes to help keep cholesterol down: magnesium, potassium, and fiber. It makes a satisfying, energy-boosting afternoon snack.

- Omega-3 fatty acids have the uncanny ability to break down cholesterol in the lining of blood vessels, as well as serving as a solvent for saturated fats in the diet. The end result is less cholesterol in the body and bloodstream, and a reduced likelihood of cholesterol/heart disease complications in the future. Flaxseed oil offers the most cost-effective and beneficial method for increasing the intake of omega-3 oils in the diet. (See "And Now May We Prevent . . ." for detailed *flaxseed oil* information.)

Dr. Ray C. Wunderlich, Jr., of the Wunderlich Center for Nutritional Medicine in St. Petersburg, Florida, recommends grape seed oil (available at health food stores) as a reliable HDL (good cholesterol) increaser. Follow the dosage on the label.

‡ ANTICLOTTING MEDICATION ALERT
Broccoli and turnip greens are rich in vitamin K, the clot-promoting vitamin. If you take anticlotting medication, be aware that eating big portions of those vegetables can counteract the effects of the medicine.

‡Hemorrhoids (Piles)

Hemorrhoids, or piles, are varicose veins in or around the rectum. It is truly a pain in the anus.

Two out of every three adults have had, currently have, or will have hemorrhoids. Chances are, if you're reading this page, you are one of the two out of the three.

Along with treating your condition with natural, non-chemical remedies, here are ways of speeding up the healing process:

- Keep the bowels as clear as possible. Drink lots of fruit juices and vegetable juices. Stay away from hard-to-digest, overly processed foods: white flour, sugar, alcoholic beverages, etc.
- Do not strain or hold your breath while having a bowel movement. Make an effort to breathe evenly.
- Take a brisk walk as often as you can, especially after meals.

Heed the suggestions above as well as the ones on the following pages, and hopefully, in a few days, you'll have this problem behind you.

Take 100 mg of rutin three times a day. This has helped hemorrhoid sufferers when all else has failed.

Apply liquid lecithin directly on the hemorrhoids, once a day, until they completely disappear.

Eat a large boiled leek every day as an afternoon snack or with dinner. Eat 3 raw unprocessed almonds every day. Chew each one about fifty times.

Insert a peeled clove of garlic in the rectum right after a bowel movement. Keep it in as long as possible. Then, before bedtime, remove it and insert another peeled clove, as high as you can push it with your finger. In order to keep it in overnight, you might have to put on a T-bandage. Garlic should help reduce the swelling quite quickly. Repeat the procedure daily until you're hemorrhoid-free.

Put a cottage cheese poultice on the hemorrhoid area to help relieve pain. Change the poultice three times a day.

In a blender, put ¼ cup cranberries and use the "finely chop" setting. Place 1 tablespoon of the blended cranberries in a piece of cheesecloth and insert it in the rectum. An hour later, remove the cheesecloth insert and replace it with another tablespoon of cranberries in cheesecloth for another hour. This is a great pain reliever. By the end of two hours, you should feel much better.

Cut a peeled, raw potato in the shape of a suppository (like a bullet) and insert it in the rectum. This folk remedy has had dramatic positive results.

Add ¼ cup of witch hazel to a basin of warm water. Sit in it for at least fifteen minutes at a time, at least two times a day. Complete cures have been reported within three days.

Psychic healer Edgar Cayce recommended this exercise to a hemorrhoid sufferer:

1. Stand with feet about six inches apart. Hands at sides.
2. Raise your hands up to the ceiling.

3. Bend forward and bring your hands as close to the floor as you can.
4. Go back to the first position.

Repeat the entire procedure thirty-six times. It should take just a few minutes to do. Do it an hour after breakfast and an hour after dinner, every day until the hemorrhoids are history.

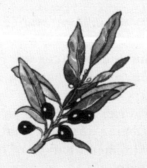

‡Hiccups

A hiccup is a spastic contraction of the diaphragm—the large circular muscle that separates the chest from the abdomen.

Hiccups are a great conversation starter. If you're in a room with thirty people, ask each one of them how they get rid of the hiccups and you will probably get thirty different remedies.

According to the *Guinness Book of World Records*, the longest recorded attack of hiccups is that which afflicted Charles Osborne of Iowa. He was born in 1894 and got the hiccups in 1922, when he was slaughtering a hog.

The hiccups continued but didn't stop him from marrying twice and fathering eight children. (Who knows, maybe it helped.)

In 1983, Guinness reported that Charles Osborne had hiccupped—and was still hiccuping—about 420 million times. By the time he died in 1990, the hiccupping had slowed down from forty times a minute to twenty times a minute. You do the math.

To prevent a case of the hiccups, do not slaughter a hog. To cure a case of the hiccups, try one or more of the following remedies.

Drink a glass of pineapple or orange juice.

Make believe your index finger is a mustache. Place it under your nose and press in hard for thirty seconds.

Drink a glass of water that has a tablespoon in it—the bowl of the spoon being the part that's in the water. As you drink, be sure the metal handle of the spoon is pressed against your left temple.

Swallow a teaspoon of fresh onion juice.

Mix a teaspoon of apple cider vinegar in a cup of warm water and drink it down.

Drink a glass of water from the far side of the glass. You have to bend far forward to do this without dribbling all over yourself.

Gently inhale a little pepper—enough to make you sneeze a couple of times. Sneezing usually makes the hiccups disappear.

Eat a piece of dry bread (a few days old, if possible). Chew each bite thoroughly. By the time you finish the slice of bread, the hiccups should be gone.

When children between the ages of seven and fourteen have the hiccups, promise to double their allowance if they can hiccup once more after you say "Go!" Chances are there will not be one more hiccup after you say "Go!" We don't know why, but it works . . . most of the time.

Place an ice cube right below the Adam's apple and count to 150.

Take a mouthful of water and keep it in your mouth while you stick the middle fingers of each hand into your ears and press fairly firmly. Count to 100, then swallow the water and unplug your ears.

Pretend you're singing at the Metropolitan Opera House without a microphone and the foremost opera critic is in the last row of the uppermost tier. One aria and the hiccups should disappear. (So might your roommate.)

Take seven drinks of water without taking a breath in between swallows. While you're drinking the water, keep turning the glass to the left.

Put a handkerchief over a glass of water and suck the water through it as you would with a straw.

Stick out your tongue as far as possible and keep it out for three minutes. Be careful, one big hiccup and—ouch!

The sole of the foot is an acupressure point for curing the hiccups. Massage the center of the sole for as long as it takes for the hiccups to stop.

Mix ½ teaspoon of sugar in ½ glass of water and drink it slowly.

Place a pencil between your teeth so that it sticks out on both sides of your mouth. Chomp down on it while drinking a glass of water.

If nothing else works, take a hot bath. This has helped cure severe cases of hiccups.

‡Indigestion

Mae West said, "Too much of a good thing is wonderful!" We say, "Too much of a good thing can cause indigestion!"

There are different types of indigestion: mild, severe, and persistent. Persistent indigestion may be a food allergy. Get professional medical help to check it out. Severe indigestion may be something a lot more serious than you think. Seek professional help immediately.

CAUTION: NEVER TAKE A LAXATIVE WHEN YOU HAVE SEVERE STOMACH PAIN.

Mild indigestion usually produces one or a combination of the following symptoms: stomachache, heartburn, nausea and vomiting, or gas.

The first thing a person suffering from a mild case of indigestion usually does is promise never to overindulge again. That takes care of next time. As for now, relief is just a page or two away.

‡ INDIGESTION IN GENERAL

By eating 1 large radish, all the symptoms and discomfort of indigestion may disappear, unless radishes do not agree with you, in which case, move on to the next remedy.

Mix 1 tablespoon of honey and 2 teaspoons of apple cider vinegar into a glass of hot water and drink the mixture.

Put on a yellow slicker, not because it's raining, but because color therapists claim that the color yellow has rays that can help heal all digestive problems. Eat yellow foods like bananas, lemons, pineapple, squash, and grapefruit. Lie down on a yellow sheet and get a massage with some yellow oil. What could be bad?

Chamomile and/or peppermint teas are very soothing. At the first sign of indigestion, drink a cup of either one.

Eat, drink, or take some form of papaya after eating. Fresh papaya (the *yellow* ones are ripe), papaya juice, or papaya pills help combat indigestion, thanks to the potent digestive enzyme papain.

In moderation, drink some white wine *after*, not during, a meal to help overcome indigestion.

Arrowroot is a wonderful stomach settler. Combine 1 tablespoon of arrowroot with enough water to make a smooth paste. Boil the mixture. Let it cool, then add 1 tablespoon of lime juice and take it when you have "agita."

Garlic helps stimulate the secretion of digestive enzymes. If you're plagued by indigestion, take garlic supplements after lunch and after dinner. Use garlic in salads and, whenever possible, in cooking, unless garlic *gives* you indigestion.

Scrub an orange and eat some of the peel five minutes after a meal.

Boiled or steamed zucchini sprinkled with raw grated almonds is a side dish with your meal that will ensure better digestion.

Cayenne pepper sprinkled sparingly (no more than ¼ teaspoon) on food or in soup will aid digestion.

Add basil to food while cooking. It will make the food more digestible and also help prevent constipation. If you really have a taste for basil, add ⅛ to ¼ teaspoon to a glass of white wine and drink it *after*, not during, the meal.

If you have trouble digesting raw vegetables, at least three hours before eating, sprinkle the veggies with fresh lemon juice. Somehow the lemon, as wild as this sounds, partly digests the hard-to-digest parts of the greens.

‡ STOMACH CRAMPS

Steep 1 teaspoon of fresh or dried parsley in 1 cup of hot water. After five minutes, strain and slowly drink the parsley tea. Remember that parsley tea also acts as a diuretic, so make sure you plan accordingly, because you may have to "eat and run."

Slice 1 medium-size onion and boil it in 1 cup of milk. Drink this concoction warm. It sounds awful and probably is, but it's an old home remedy that may work.

Water has amazing healing power. Get in a hot shower and let the water beat down on your stomach for ten to fifteen minutes. By the time you dry off, you should be feeling a lot better.

American Indians used this one for stomachaches: Pour 1 cup of boiling water over 1 teaspoon of cornmeal. Let it sit for five minutes. Add salt to taste and drink slowly.

‡ NAUSEA AND VOMITING

Always keep a bottle of ginger ale in the refrigerator. When you feel nauseous, drink about ½ cup of the soda. One or two burps later, you'll feel fine again.

Drink a cup of chamomile tea to calm the stomach and stop vomiting.

A couple of cloves steeped in boiling water for five minutes may do the trick, after you've drunk it, of course. If the taste of cloves reminds you too much of the dentist, then steep a piece of cinnamon stick in boiling water, or 1 teaspoon of powdered ginger. All of them are fine for stopping nausea and vomiting.

Crack an ice cube and suck on the little pieces. It's worth a try when you have nothing else in the house.

This remedy is the pits—the armpits. Peel a large onion and cut it in half. Place each half under each armpit. As nauseating as it sounds, we've been told it stops vomiting and relieves nausea in no time.

If you're outside, feeling nauseous, stop at the nearest luncheonette and ask for a teaspoon of pure cola syrup with a water chaser.

If you're home and have cola soda or even root beer, let it go flat by stirring it. Once the fizz is gone, drink 2 or 3 ounces to ease the nausea.

‡ HEARTBURN

Whatever you do, don't lie down when you have heartburn. Instead, stay on your feet and try one of the following:

Eat six blanched almonds. Chew each one at least thirty times.

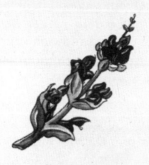

Eat a slice of raw potato.

Or: Grate a raw potato and put it in cheesecloth. Squeeze out the juice in a glass. Add twice the amount of warm water as potato juice and drink it down.

Mix 1 tablespoon of apple cider vinegar and 1 tablespoon of honey into a cup of warm water. Stir and drink.

Peel and eat a raw carrot. Chew each bite thirty times.

If you have heartburn from eating something sweet, squeeze ½ lemon into a cup of warm water. Add ½ teaspoon of salt and drink it slowly.

‡ GAS/FLATULENCE

A strong cup of peppermint tea will give you relief quickly, especially if you walk around as you drink it.

A hot water compress placed directly on the stomach can relieve gas pains.

Add 1 teaspoon of anisette liqueur to a cup of warm water. Stir and sip.

An old home remedy for gas and heartburn is a raw onion sandwich. Some people would rather *have* gas and heartburn than eat a raw onion sandwich, and some people *get* gas and heartburn from a raw onion sandwich. If onions agree with you, it's worth a try.

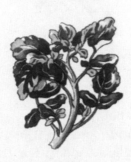

This gas-expelling yoga technique should be done in the privacy of your bedroom. Lie on the bed facedown with one leg tucked under you. Got the picture? Your knee is under your chest. Stay that way for three or four minutes, then stretch out that leg and bring the other leg up, with the knee under your chest. Every three or four minutes reverse the legs. Stop when you've expelled the gas.

Add ½ teaspoon of bay leaves to a cup of boiling water. Let it steep, then strain it and drink it down slowly.

Get rid of a gas condition with mustard seeds and lots of water. The first day take 2 seeds; the second day take 4 and so on until you take 12 seeds on the sixth day. Then work it down to 2 seeds on the eleventh day. By then you should be fine. Continue to take 2 seeds a day. Always take the mustard seeds on an empty stomach.

‡ BELCHING

This is a Taoist remedy that dates back to the sixth century B.C. Scrub a tangerine, then peel it and boil the pieces of peel for five minutes. Strain, let cool, and drink the tangerine tea. The tea should stop you from belching. You can also eat the tangerine peel as a digestive aid.

‡Infants and Children

Every baby-care book tells you to "childproof" your home. Make a crawling tour of each room in your house in order to see things from a child's-eye view. Once you're aware of the danger zones, you can eliminate them by covering wires, nailing down furniture, etc. Do this every four to six months as the child grows and is able to reach more things.

Still, no matter how childproof a place is, a mishap can happen. We suggest that parents have a first-aid book handy and/or take a first-aid course through the local American Red Cross.

It's also very important to keep a list of the following emergency numbers near every telephone in the house:
• Pediatrician
• Poison Control Center
• Police
• Fire Department
• Hospital
• Pharmacy
• Dentist
• Neighbors (with cars)

In terms of home remedies for common conditions, we caution you that children's systems are much more delicate than ours. So, while lots of the remedies throughout the book can certainly be applied to youngsters, use good common sense in prescribing doses and strengths. In all cases, check with the pediatrician first.

One major caution: NEVER GIVE HONEY TO A CHILD UNDER ONE YEAR OLD! Spores found in honey have been linked to botulism in babies.

Here are some remedies specifically for children's

ailments. They should help you as well as your child to get through those tough times.

‡ BEDWETTING

Give the bedwetter a few pieces of cinnamon bark to chew on throughout the day. For some unknown reason, it seems to control bedwetting for some kids.

Prepare a cup of corn silk tea by adding 10 to 15 drops of corn silk extract to a cup of boiled water. Stir, let cool, and have the bedwetter slowly sip the tea right before bedtime.

If all else fails, try this: At bedtime, tie a towel around the bedwetter's loins, making sure the knot is in front. This urges the child to sleep on his or her back, which seems to lessen bedwetting urges.

NOTE: Chronic bedwetters should be treated by a health professional.

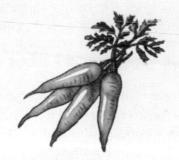

‡ CINDER IN EYE

Irrigate eye with water.

Peel an onion near the child so that tears wash away the cinder.

‡ COUGH

When a child has a bad, hacking cough, spray the pillow with wine vinegar. Both you and the child may sleep better for it.

‡ DIAPER RASH

Let baby's bottom be exposed to the air. If weather permits, the sun (ten to fifteen minutes at a time) can do wonders for clearing up diaper rash.

Gently apply honey to the rash. It helps promote healing.

‡ DIARRHEA

Give baby pure blackberry juice.
DOSE: 2 or 3 tablespoons four times a day.

Carrot soup not only soothes the inflamed small bowel, it also replaces lost body fluids and minerals. Also carrots have an antidiarrheal substance called pectin. You can prepare the soup by mixing a jar of strained carrots baby food with a jar of water. Feed the child carrot soup as long as diarrhea persists.

Another way of treating diarrhea in infants is to give them barley water throughout the day. (See "Preparation Guide" for the barley water recipe.)

‡ FEVER

To help pull down a child's fever, put sliced, raw potatoes on the soles of the feet and bandage in place. Let the novelty of this remedy provide a few laughs for you and your child. Isn't laughter the best medicine?

Give your child a long, soothing bath in tepid water. Then, when you tuck your child in, be sure the blanket is not tucked in too tight. Leave it loose so that the heat can escape into the air.

‡ HICCUPS
When our friend's six-month-old girl gets the hiccups, Daddy yells at the dog. That makes baby cry. As soon as the baby takes her first deep breath to cry, Daddy quickly cups his hands over her ears and the hiccups stop. (If his dog gets the hiccups, we wonder if he yells at his baby.)

‡ INDIGESTION, COLIC, AND GAS
Give your colicky infant mild ginger tea. It's wonderful for digestion and gas problems.

For fifteen minutes, boil a cup of water with ⅓ of a bay leaf in the water. Let it cool, then pour it into the baby's bottle and let the baby drink it. This old Sicilian remedy has cured many colicky bambinos.

Mild chamomile tea will soothe an upset stomach and calm down colicky kids. That is, if you can calm them down long enough to drink the chamomile tea.

If your child seems to have a minor digestion problem, try 2 teaspoons of apple juice concentrate in half a glass of water before meals. Make sure the liquid mixture is room temperature, not chilled.

‡ PIGEON-TOES
If your child is slightly pigeon-toed, buy a pair of shoes one size larger than he or she usually takes. Have the child

wear them to bed every night with the right shoe on the left foot and the left shoe on the right foot. If there is no improvement within a reasonable amount of time, obviously your child will need more sophisticated treatment.

‡ HEAD LICE

It's estimated that at any given time, ten million Americans have head lice. Lice are transmitted from child to child via a common headrest, like a mat in the school gymnasium, or from a seat at the movies. Just about the only way you could prevent a child from ever being exposed to lice is by keeping that child in a bubble. Since the bubble is not an option, should your child have lice, know that there are over-the-counter shampoos that are safe and effective, unlike the prescription shampoos that can be dangerous to young children, pregnant or nursing women, and anyone with a cut on her hand or arm. A friend tried several over-the-counter shampoos and found that the safest one that worked best on her child's head was Rid.

For shampoo to be effective, leave it on the child's head for at least five minutes; ten minutes is even better.

‡ NIT-PICKING

After you shampoo and get rid of the lice, make sure you get rid of any remaining nits (eggs or young lice) by thoroughly rinsing with equal parts of white vinegar and water. Or first you can comb tea tree oil (available at health food stores) through the hair, and then rinse with vinegar and water.

CAUTION: Do not use your fingers to hunt down these critters; they can burrow their way under your fingernails. Yuck!

‡ EYELASH NITS

If the nits move down to the eyelashes, DO NOT use tea tree oil. It's much too strong and dangerous near the eyes. Instead, before breakfast and after supper, carefully put a thin layer of petroleum jelly on the lashes. Do this for eight days. By then, the jelly will have smothered the nits and you will be able to simply remove them.

‡ SPITTING UP

Warm up a little heavy syrup from canned peaches and give it to your baby to stop nausea.

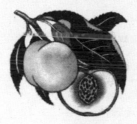

‡ SPLINTERS

To pinpoint the exact location of a splinter, pat some iodine on the area and the sliver of wood will absorb it and turn dark.

Once you've located the splinter, soak the area in vegetable oil for three minutes or as long as the child will stay in one place. The oil should allow the splinter to glide right out.

If the child has a sliver of glass, numb the area with an ice cube or some teething lotion before you start the painful squeezing and scraping.

‡ TEETHING

When teething children are being fed, they often cry as though they do not want the food. They may really be hungry but be crying because of the pain caused by a metal spoon. Feed the teething tot with an ivory, wood, or bone spoon and make sure the edges are nice and smooth.

Rub the sore little gums with olive oil to help relieve the pain.

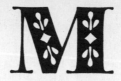

‡Male Problems

It is estimated that one out of every three men over the age of sixty has some kind of prostate problem.

We strongly suggest that if you are suffering with pain, burning, testicular or scrotal swelling, or any other prostate-related symptoms, you have your condition evaluated by a health professional.

As for impotence, most men at some time during their lives experience the dreaded inability to have an erection. That's the bad news. The good news is that it is usually a temporary condition commonly caused nowadays by prescription drugs or by some kind of psychological trauma and emotional tension. While the psyche is being treated with professional help, physical steps can be taken to improve one's sexual energy.

You might want to read through these health hints whether or not anything is bothering you. Chances are you'll find some information you can use to help you maintain your health and sexual potency.

‡ PROSTATE

The prostate contains ten times more zinc than most other organs in the body. Pumpkin seeds have a very high zinc content. That may account for the normalizing effect it is said the seeds have on prostate disorders. It may also be beneficial because of the seeds' iron, phosphorus, vitamins A and B_1, protein, calcium, and unsaturated fatty acid content. For whatever reason, pumpkin seeds might have a positive effect on the male genital system.

Eat three or four palmsful (about ½ cup) of unprocessed (unsalted) shelled pumpkin seeds daily. If you can't get pumpkin seeds, sunflower seeds are second best. Or take zinc tablets—15 mg two times a day. For chronic prostate trouble, take 50 mg a day for six months, then reduce the dosage to 30 mg a day.

NOTE: All of these prostate remedies should be used with professional medical supervision.

Bee pollen is said to be effective in reducing swelling of the prostate as well as treating other prostate disorders. Pollen contains the hormone testosterone and traces of other male hormones. It seems to give the prostate a boost so that it may heal itself.

DOSE: 5 pollen pills daily—2 in the morning, 2 in the afternoon, and 1 in the evening (or the equivalent in bee pollen granules).

Drink 2 to 4 ounces of coconut milk every day to tone up the prostate glands. The milk is pure and uncontaminated and loaded with minerals. It's also a soothing digestive aid. (See "Preparation Guide" for instructions on milking a coconut.)

When the prostate gland is inflamed, apply a watercress poultice to reduce the inflammation.

To relieve prostate pain, in a circular motion, massage the area above the heel and just below the inner ankle of each foot and/or the inside of the wrists, above the palm of each hand. Keep massaging until the pain and soreness disappear.

Prepare parsley tea by steeping a handful of fresh parsley in a cup of hot water for ten minutes. Drink a few cups of tea throughout the day.

Take hot sitz baths—two a day. Sit in half a foot of hot water for about fifteen minutes. Within a week, inflammation and swelling should be greatly reduced.

Corn silk tea has been a popular folk remedy for prostate problems. Steep a handful of the silky strings that grow around ears of corn in a cup of hot water for ten minutes. Drink a few cups throughout the day. If it's not fresh corn season, buy corn silk extract in health food stores, and add 10 to 15 drops in 1 cup of water and drink.

‡ SCROTUM AND TESTICLES

A comfrey poultice applied to the scrotum might reduce swelling and soreness. (See "Poultices" in the "Preparation Guide.")

To relieve testicle pain, massage the outer wrist of each hand and/or the outer ankle of each foot.

‡ MALE PROBLEMS IN GENERAL

To relax tension, stimulate circulation, and generally soothe the male organs, massage the area behind the leg in back of the ankle, about one or two inches higher than the shoe line of each foot.

Don't forget that nearly everything works better when it's used. Many men enjoy better urination by seeing to it that appropriate ejaculation occurs on a regular basis.

‡ IMPOTENCE

According to the teachings of Yogi Bhajan, a man should never have sexual intercourse within two and a half hours after eating a meal, the length of time it takes to digest food.

The sex act is strenuous and requires your mind, your entire nervous system, and all your muscles needed for the digestion process. Yogi Bhajan felt that lovemaking right after eating could ruin your stomach and, if done often, could eventually result in premature ejaculation.

While he said that four hours between eating and sex is adequate, he thought that for optimal sexual function, a man should have nothing but liquids and juices twenty-four hours before making love.

Garlic is said to stimulate sexual desire and the production of semen. Eat raw garlic in salads and use it in cooking and take 2 garlic pills a day. Then find a woman who doesn't mind the smell of garlic. By the way, is it a coincidence that the French and Italians have a steady diet of garlic and are said to be vigorous lovers?

Mint is supposed to restore sexual desire. Eat mint leaves and drink mint tea. It's also good for garlic breath.

In Japan, men are advised to firmly squeeze their testicles daily, once for as many years as they are old.

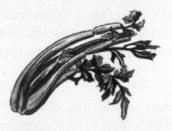

After much research, we've come up with a list of foods said to have aphrodisiacal effects. At the top of the list is, believe it or not, celery. Eat it every day. Of course, we've

all heard about eating oysters. Do! BUT BEWARE OF CON-
TAMINATED SOURCES! Oysters contain zinc and, like pumpkin seeds, are said to be wonderful for male genitalia. The
list continues with peaches, honey, parsley, cayenne pepper, bran cereals, and truffles. In fact, Napoleon credited
truffles for his ability to sire a son.

American Indians used ginseng as an aphrodisiac. The
Chinese also use ginseng. This herb should be taken sparingly, about ¼ teaspoon twice a month. It is said to stimulate the endocrine system and be a source of male
hormones. Ginseng has also been said to help men who
have had a sterility problem.

Contrary to what we've been led to believe about cold
showers, they might help stimulate sexual desire. Every day
for about two months, take a cold shower or cold sitz bath
and notice a rejuvenated you.

NOTE: If you have prostate problems, take *hot* sitz baths.

To improve sexual potency, do this yoga exercise before
breakfast and before bedtime: Sit on the floor with back
straight, head up, and feet crossed in front of you. Tighten
the muscles in the genital area, including the anus. Count
to twenty, then relax and count to twenty again. Repeat the
procedure five times in a row, twice a day.

The English have a commercial preparation called Tonic
for Happy Lovers. The recipe consists of combining 1 ounce
of licorice root with 2 teaspoons of crushed fennel seeds
(both of which you should be able to get at a health food
store) and 2 cups of water. Bring the mixture to a boil,
lower the heat, cover, and simmer slowly for twenty minutes. After it has cooled, strain it and bottle it.

DOSE: 1 to 3 tablespoons twice a day.

NOTE: If you have high blood pressure, do not take licorice root.

‡Memory

There seems to be a national epidemic of memory failure. Lately, I hear people of all ages saying things like "I don't remember a thing anymore." "I feel as though I'm losing my mind." "The only thing my memory is good for is to make me wonder what I've forgotten."

There's a vitamin store on the Upper East Side of New York City where the sales clerk offers two bottles of Maximum Memory pills at a reduced rate. He also gives you a money-back guarantee if, after finishing the first bottle of pills, your memory hasn't greatly improved. Everyone buys two bottles of pills. That's super salesmanship. Think about it. If, after you finish the first bottle, your memory does improve, you will want to keep taking the pills and not return the second bottle. On the other hand, if your memory is still as bad after you've taken the first bottle, chances are you won't remember the salesman's offer, or the place you bought the pills.

It's sort of the same with this chapter. If these memory remedies help, fine. If not, hopefully you won't remember where you've heard about them.

Choline is used by our brains to make the important chemical acetylcholine, which is required for memory.

At a health food or vitamin store, buy choline chloride or choline hydrochloride, *not* choline bitartrate. (The latter sometimes causes diarrhea.) Taking choline may improve your memory and your ability to learn. You should also notice a keener sense of mental organization.

DOSE: Take 500 mg of choline twice a day. (Set your alarm clock so you won't forget to take it.)

A memory-improving drink: half a glass of carrot juice together with half a glass of milk, daily.

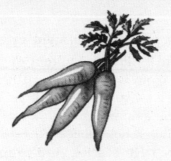

Three prunes a day supposedly improves the memory. It can also help prevent constipation, and since constipation paralyzes the thinking process, take 3 prunes a day.

Daily doses of fresh ginger used in cooking and for tea may heighten the memory.

Add 4 cloves to a cup of sage tea. Sage and cloves have been said to strengthen the memory. Drink a cup every day.

‡Motion Sickness

‡ MOTION SICKNESS IN GENERAL

The story is told about the captain of the ship who announced, "There is no hope. We are all doomed. The ship is sinking and we'll all be dead within an hour." One voice was heard after the announcement. It was the seasick passenger saying, "Thank heavens!"

If you have ever been seasick, you probably anticipated that punchline.

Most people think air, land, and sea sickness start in the stomach. WRONG! Guess again. Constant jarring of the semicircular canals in the ears cause inner balance problems that produce those awful motion sickness symptoms. What to do? Go suck a lemon! Really! That's one of the time-tested remedies. There are a few more that might help you get through that miserable feeling.

Before there's a "next time," be sure to read the "And Now May We Prevent . . ." chapter, as well as this one.

Pull out and pinch the skin in the middle of your inner wrist, about an inch from your palm. Keep pulling and pinching alternate wrists until you feel better.

A cup of peppermint or chamomile tea may calm down the stomach and alleviate nausea.

Mix ⅛ teaspoon of cayenne pepper in a cup of warm water or a cup of soup and force yourself to finish it, even if you think it'll finish you. It won't. But it may stop the nausea.

At the first sign of motion sickness, take a metal comb or wire brush and run the teeth over the backs of your hands, particularly the area from the thumb to the first finger, including the web of skin in between both fingers. You may have relief in five to ten minutes.

Briskly massage the fourth and fifth fingers of each hand, with particular emphasis on the vicinity of the pinky's knuckle. You may feel relief within fifteen minutes; if not, go suck a lemon!

During a bout of motion sickness, suck a lemon or drink some fresh-squeezed lemon juice.

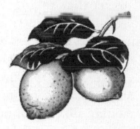

‡ JET LAG—TRAVEL PLAN CONSIDERATIONS

Generally, it takes a day to recover for each time zone you pass through. New York to California: three time zones, three days of jet lag. Actually, going east to west and gaining a few hours is better jet-lag-wise than west to east when you lose a few hours.

In terms of getting that first good night's sleep at your destination, it seems best to plan on arriving in the evening. England's Royal Air Force Institute of Aviation Medicine suggests: When flying east, fly early; when heading west, fly late.

Surely you've heard that alcohol is one of the most powerful dehydrators there is. And you must know that just being in an airplane is dehydrating. But do you know that dehydration makes jet lag worse? Conclusion: *Do not drink any alcoholic beverages while airborne.* Do drink lots of water and juice—as much as possible. If you have to keep going to the lavatory, good. Walking up and down the aisles will help refresh and prepare you for your new time zone.

‡ JET LAG PREVENTION

A couple of days before flying, take ginkgo-hawthorn tincture (available at health food stores) and follow the dosage on the label.

It's been reported to us that taking ½ to 1 mg of melatonin right before boarding the plane has prevented jet lag. If you know that you really suffer from jet lag, ask your doctor about taking melatonin before your upcoming flight. The jury doesn't seem to be in on melatonin yet. Some studies in animals suggest that people with high blood pressure or cardiovascular disease should not take melatonin. Again, consult with your health professional before taking it.

‡Sciatica

Sciatica is a painful condition affecting the sciatic nerve, which is the longest nerve in the body. It extends from the lower spine through the pelvis, thighs, down into the legs and ends at the heels.

We all have some nerve!

The home remedies we describe may not cure the condition, but they may help ease the pain.

The juice from potatoes has been said to help sciatic sufferers. So has celery juice. If you don't have a juicer, your local health food store, one with a juice bar, might be willing to accommodate you. Have them juice a 10-ounce combination of potato and celery juice. Add carrots and/or beets to improve the taste. In addition to the juice, drink a couple of cups of celery tea throughout the day.

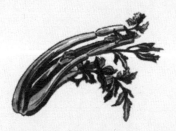

Stimulate the nerve by applying a fresh minced horseradish poultice to the painful area. Keep it on for one hour.

According to the *Pakistan Medical Times*, vitamin B_1 and garlic are very beneficial. Eat garlic raw in salads and use it in cooking. Also, take garlic supplements daily, plus 10 mg of vitamin B_1 along with a good vitamin B complex.

A hot water bag on the painful area may help you make it through the night with less pain and more sleep.

Drink elderberry juice and elderberry tea throughout the day.

Before bedtime, heat olive oil and use it to massage the painful areas.

Eat lots of watercress and parsley every day.

‡Skin

Skin is the largest organ of the body. The average adult has seventeen square feet of skin. Thick or thin skinned, it weighs about five pounds.

Five pounds of skin covering seventeen square feet of body surface . . . that's a lot of room for eruptions, cuts, sores, grazes, scrapes, scratches, and itches.

Someone named Anonymous once said, "Dermatology is the best specialty. The patient never dies—and never gets well."

Mr. Anonymous said that before reading this chapter.

‡ PIMPLES

Mix the juice of 2 garlic cloves with an equal amount of vinegar and dab it on the pimples every evening. The condition may clear up in a couple of weeks.

Simmer 1 sliced medium onion in ½ cup of honey until the onion is soft. Then mash the mixture into a smooth paste. Make sure it's cool before applying it to blemishes. Leave it on at least one hour, then rinse off with warm water. Repeat procedure every evening until "Look Ma, no pimples!"

Eat brown rice regularly. It contains amino acids that are good for skin conditions.

About four hours before bedtime, steep 1 cup of mashed strawberries in 2 cups (1 pint) of white vinegar. Let it steep until you're ready for bed. Then strain the pulp and seeds. Massage the remaining liquid on your face and have a good night's sleep. It's not as messy as it sounds. The liquid dries on the face before the face touches the pillow. In the morning, wash it off with cool water. This is an excellent cleanser and astringent for blemished skin.

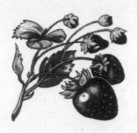

‡ BLACKHEADS

Before going to bed, rub lemon juice over blackheads. Wait until morning to wash off the juice with cool water. Repeat procedure several evenings in a row and you'll see big improvement in the skin.

‡ ACNE

Wet a clean, white cloth or towel with your fresh, warm, first urine of the day and pat it on the acne areas. Better than your own urine is the less-polluted urine of a baby. If you have access to an infant's wet diaper, apply it to the affected areas and you'll see amazing results within a short period of time.

Compared to the urine remedy for acne, this solution may be easier to take, but it's harder to make. Combine 4 ounces of grated horseradish with a pint of 90-proof alcohol. Add a pinch of grated nutmeg and a chopped up bitter orange peel available at herb and health food stores. With sterilized cotton, dab some of this solution on each pimple every morning and every evening.

‡ ACNE SCARS

To help remove acne scars, combine 1 teaspoon of powdered nutmeg with 1 teaspoon of honey and apply it to the scarred area. After twenty minutes, wash it off with cool water. Do this twice a week, and hopefully within a couple of months you will see an improvement.

‡ BLOTCHY, SCALY, AND ITCHY SKIN (SEBORRHEA)

Apply cod-liver oil to blotchy, scaly, and itchy skin. Leave it on as long as possible. When you finally wash it off, use cool water. Health food stores now carry nonsmelly, Norwegian, emulsified cod-liver oil.

Rub on some liquid lecithin and leave it on the problem skin areas as long as possible. Use cool water to wash it off. Repeat the procedure as often as possible . . . several times a day.

‡ DEAD SKIN CELLS AND ENLARGED PORES

A friend of ours uses Miracle Whip salad dressing to remove dead skin cells and to tighten her pores. She puts it on her face and leaves it there for about twenty minutes. Then she washes it off with warm water, followed by cold water. She claims that no other mayonnaise works as well as Miracle Whip salad dressing. Maybe that's where the "Miracle" comes in.

Papaya contains the enzyme papain, which is said to do wonderful things for the complexion. Wash your face and neck. Remove the meat of the papaya (it makes a delicious lunch) and rub the inside of the papaya skin on your skin. It will dry, forming a see-through mask. After fifteen minutes, wash it off with warm water. Along with removing dead skin and tightening the pores, it may make some light freckles disappear.

‡ EXTRA-LARGE ENLARGED PORES

We're talking really big pores here. Every night for one week, or as long as one container of buttermilk lasts, wash your face, then soak a wad of absorbent cotton in buttermilk and dab it all over your face. After twenty minutes, smile. It's a very weird sensation. Wash the dried buttermilk off with cool water.

NOTE: The smile is optional.

‡ ROUGH AND TOUGH DEAD SKIN CELLS

Make a paste by combining salt and lemon juice. Rub this abrasive mixture on rough and tough areas such as elbows, feet, and knees. Wash the paste off with cool water.

‡ MASK FOR DRY SKIN

Scrub 2 to 3 medium-size carrots, cut each carrot in 1-inch pieces, and put them in a pot with a few cups of water. Cook the carrots until they are slightly softened. Transfer the carrots to a blender or food processor and puree. Distribute the carrot puree all over your just-washed face and neck. Keep it there for about twenty minutes, then rinse with tepid water. This mask is popular in European spas, where continual use is said to improve elasticity as well as smooth out wrinkles.

‡ MASK FOR OILY SKIN

Kitty litter has great absorbency and can be used for lots of things, including the purr-fect facial for oily skin. Be sure to get a natural litter that's 100 percent clay, no chemicals added. Mash 2 tablespoons of the litter with enough water—about an ounce—to make it paste consistency. Apply it to your just-washed face, but not to the delicate area around your eyes. Leave it on for about fifteen minutes. Rinse off with tepid water.

‡ MASK FOR ALL SKIN TYPES

In a blender, puree 1 cup of fresh pineapple and ½ cup of fresh (slightly green) papaya. Put the pureed fruit in a bowl and mix in 2 tablespoons of honey. Apply it to your just-washed face and neck, but not on the delicate area around your eyes. Leave it on for five minutes, not more, and rinse with cool water. This once-a-week alpha hydroxy facial can boost the production of collagen (making your face firmer), slough off dead skin cells, even out skin tone, and make tiny lines less noticeable. The enzymes in pineapple (bromelain) and papaya (papain) do most of the work as the honey hydrates the skin.

‡ SKIN TONER

In a blender, puree 4 medium-size, well-washed strawberries, 2 dollops of plain yogurt, and a tablespoon of freshly squeezed lemon juice. Distribute the strawberry puree all over your face and neck. Leave it on for about twenty minutes, then rinse with tepid water. Doing this skin toning treatment twice a week is said to help prevent little age lines.

‡ PSORIASIS

A cabin at the shore and frequent dips in the surf or a trip to Israel's Dead Sea seems to work wonders for psoriasis sufferers. Next best thing: Dissolve ½ cup of sea salt in

1 gallon of water. Soak the psoriasis patches in the sea salt water several times a day—whenever possible.

Foremost authority on healing herbs Dr. James Duke explains in *The Green Pharmacy*, "Several plant oils are chemically similar to fish oils, which have a reputation for helping to relieve psoriasis. Flaxseed oil contains the beneficial compounds eicosapentaenoic acid and alpha-linolenic acid." Dr. Duke reviewed studies showing that 10 to 12 grams (5 to 6 teaspoons) of flaxseed oil can help treat psoriasis. (See "And Now May We Prevent . . ." for more details on flaxseed oil and the way to take it.)

Every evening, pat garlic oil on the affected area, by puncturing a garlic soft gel and squishing out the oil. It may help clear up the condition.

‡ ECZEMA

I've been told that eating raw potatoes—at least 2 a day—has worked miracles in clearing up eczema. If you don't see an improvement after a couple of weeks, try something else.

NOTE: Persistent or chronic psoriasis and eczema conditions are best treated by a health professional.

‡ PAPER CUTS

Clean the cut with the juice of a lemon. Then, to ease the pain, wet the cut finger and dip it into powdered cloves. Since cloves act as a mild anesthetic, the pain should be gone in a matter of seconds.

‡ WEEPING SORES (INFECTIONS WITH PUS)

Place a piece of papaya pulp on a weeping sore. Keep it in place with a big Band-Aid. Change the dressing every two to three hours until it clears up.

Dab on lavender oil throughout the day. It should help heal the sore, and also help you relax.

Apply a poultice of either raw, grated carrots or cooked, mashed carrots to stop the throbbing and draw out the infection.

A honey poultice is disinfecting and healing. Use raw unprocessed honey.

NOTE: If infection persists, consult a health professional.

‡ BRUISES

If you close a door or drawer on your finger, prepare a poultice of grated onion and salt and apply it to the bruised area. The pain will disappear within seconds.

Place ice on a bruise to help prevent the area from turning black and blue, and to reduce the swelling. If ice is not available, immediately press a knife (flat side only—we're talking bruises, not amputation) or a spoon on the bruise for five to ten minutes.

Make a salve by mashing pieces of parsley into a teaspoon of butter. Gently rub the salve on the bruise.

‡ SCRATCHES, SMALL CUTS, AND GRAZES

The first thing to do when you get a scratch, small cut, or graze is to rinse it with water. Put honey on the opening and let its enzymes heal you.

Put the inside of a banana peel directly on the wound and secure it in place with an Ace bandage. Change the peel every three to four hours. We've seen remarkable and rapid results with banana peels. Carry bananas when you go camping.

‡ BLEEDING WOUNDS

If the wound is bleeding quite profusely, apply direct pressure, preferably with a sterile dressing, and seek medical attention immediately.

If the bleeding is not severe, the following remedies may help:

Lemon is an effective disinfectant and also stops a cut from bleeding. Squeeze some juice on the cut and get ready for the sting.

Sprinkle on some cayenne pepper or black pepper to stop the flow of blood from a cut within seconds. Put it directly on the cut. Yes, it will sting.

A clump of wet tobacco will stop the bleeding. So will a wet cigarette paper.

Cobwebs on an open wound stop the bleeding instantly. In fact, they are so good at clotting a wound that they've been used for years on cows right after they've been de-horned. However, all kinds of bacteria carried by the cobwebs might infect the open wound. Use cobwebs only when there is absolutely nothing else to use—like the next time you get a gash in a haunted house.

The crushed leaves of a geranium plant applied to the cut act as a styptic pencil and stop the bleeding.

‡ FINGER SORES (WHITLOWS)

When you have one of those painful inflammations around the fingernail, soak it in hot water. Then heat a lemon in the oven, cut a narrow opening in the middle, and sprinkle salt in it. Take the infected finger and stick it in the lemon. Within minutes, the pain should disappear.

‡ BOILS

Slowly heat 1 cup of milk. Just as slowly, add 3 teaspoons of salt as the milk gets close to boiling. Once the salt has been added, take the milk off the heat and add flour to thicken the mixture and to make a poultice. Apply it to the boil. The heat of the poultice will help bring it to a head, but be careful that it's not too hot.

Gently peel off the skin of a hard-boiled egg. Wet that delicate membrane and place it on the boil. It should draw pus out and relieve the inflammation.

Apply fresh slices of pumpkin to the boil. Renew the slices often until the boil comes to a head.

A poultice of cooked, minced garlic or raw chopped garlic applied to the boil will draw out the infection.

Heat a lemon in the oven, then slice it in half and place the inside part of one half on the boil. Secure it in place for about one hour.

"And Isaiah said, 'Take a lump of figs.' And they took and laid it on the boil, and he recovered."
—2 Kings 20:7.

Roast a fresh fig. Cut it in half and lay the mushy inner part on the boil. Secure it in place for a couple of hours. Then warm the other half of the roasted fig and replace the first half with it. And thou shalt recover when the boil runneth over.

‡ WHEN THE BOIL BREAKS

The boil is at the brink of breaking when it turns red and the pain increases. When it finally does break, pus will be expelled, leaving a big hole in the skin. Almost magically, the pain will disappear. Boil 1 cup of water and add 2 tablespoons of lemon juice. Let it cool. Clean and disinfect the area thoroughly with the lemon water. Cover with a sterile bandage. For the next few days, two or three times a day, remove the bandage and apply a warm, wet compress, leaving it on for fifteen minutes. Re-dress the area with a fresh sterile bandage.

‡ POISON IVY

At least one of the three poison weeds—ivy, oak, and sumac—grows in just about every state of the United States. They all produce the same sort of uncomfortable reactions. Chances are, if you're allergic to one, you're allergic to all. It's estimated that as many as ten million Americans are affected by these plants.

This may be a little *iffy*, but . . . *If* you know you're going into poison-ivy territory, and *if* it's green-tomato season, take green tomatoes with you. The second you know that poison ivy sap is on your skin, cut up the tomato and squeeze the juice on the affected area. It may save you the anguish of having poison ivy.

Once you have the poison ivy rash, use a mixture of equal parts of white vinegar and rubbing alcohol. Dab the solution on each time the itching starts. It should relieve the itching and, at the same time, dry up the rash.

Mash a piece of white chalk so that it's powdery. Then mix the powder in a pint of water. With a clean cloth, apply the mixture onto the poison ivy parts. Repeat the procedure several times a day. This is an especially convenient cure for schoolteachers.

Rub the inside of a banana skin directly on the sore skin, using a fresh banana skin every hour for a full day.

Take the leftover bananas, cut them into 2-inch pieces, put them in a plastic bag, and freeze them. They're great as an ingredient in a smoothie, along with a couple of strawberries, a dollop of yogurt, and 10 ounces of pineapple juice. Or blend frozen banana pieces in a high-powered blender until the mixture is the consistency of soft ice cream and have it as a delicious, low-calorie dessert. On a hot day, it's refreshing to munch on plain frozen banana pieces.

Apply fresh mud to the infected areas. At the end of each day, shower the mud off (not that we have to tell you to do that). Keep up this daily procedure until the redness caused by poison ivy disappears.

Slice 1 or 2 lemons and rub them all over your affected areas. It should stop the itching and help clear up the skin.

Chop 4 cloves of garlic and boil them in 1 cup of water. After the mixture cools, apply it with a clean cloth to the poison ivy areas. Repeat often—but that's the way it is with garlic . . . repeating often.

If none of the poison ivy remedies work and you're stuck with it—its usual duration is about ten days—then rub on four-leaf clovers, and have a "rash of good luck!"

‡ SPLINTERS

Boil water, then carefully fill a wide-mouthed bottle to within half an inch of the top. Place the splintered part of the finger over the top of the bottle and lightly press down. The pressing should allow the heat to draw out the splinter.

If the splintered finger is very sore, tape a slice of raw onion around the area and leave it on overnight. The swelling and the splinter should be gone by morning.

Make a paste of oatmeal, banana, and a little water and apply it to the splintered area. Alternate it with salad oil compresses, and by the end of the day, you should be able to squeeze out the splinter.

‡ BLISTERS

The fastest and easiest way to do away with a blister is to have a snail crawl over it. We don't know if this remedy really works, although we have heard it from several reliable sources. If you have a blister and you have a snail . . . let us know.

‡ SHINGLES

For relief from a painful case of shingles, prepare a paste of Epsom salts and water. Place the paste directly on the affected area. Repeat the procedure as often as possible.

Apply any of the following to relieve the itching and speed the healing: witch hazel (an astringent), apple cider vinegar (an infection fighter), red raspberry tea (particularly good for viral eruptive problems), or aloe vera gel.

‡ ITCHING (PRURITIS)

'TIS BETTER THAN RICHES TO SCRATCH WHEN IT ITCHES!

For relief, apply any one of the following to your itchy areas:
- Fresh sliced carrots
- 1 vitamin C tablet dissolved in 1 cup of warm water
- Lemon juice (for genital areas, dilute the juice)
- Raw onion slices
- A paste of uncooked oatmeal with a little water
- Apple cider vinegar (for genital areas or areas near the eyes, use diluted apple cider vinegar)

If you're itching to bathe, add 2 cups of apple cider vinegar to the bathwater, or add 3 tablespoons of baking soda to your bathwater, or add a pint of thyme tea to your bathwater. Thyme has thymol, an antiseptic, antibacterial substance that can make your itch disappear.

If you prefer a shower to a bath, take a real-quick shower under hot water—as hot as you can manage without burning yourself. The hot water has been known to stop the itching for hours at a time. I recently had an itchy patch on my back. The way I found relief was by taking a fast, hot shower and for a few seconds before ending the shower, I let the c-c-c-c-cold water run on my back. It stopped the itching, and I was able to sleep through the night. See what works best for you.

NOTE: None of the above offer relief from the Seven-Year Itch.

‡ RECTAL ITCHING

Soak a cotton pad in apple cider vinegar and place it on affected itching area. If the area is raw from scratching, be prepared for a temporary burning sensation. Leave the soaked cotton pad on overnight. (You can keep it in place with a sanitary napkin.) You should have instant relief. If itching starts again during the day, repeat the procedure instead of scratching.

Before bedtime, take a shower, then pat dry the itchy area and apply wheat germ oil. To avoid messy bedclothes and linens, put a sanitary napkin over the oily area.

‡ ITCHING FROM HIVES

Form a paste by mixing cream of tartar and water. Apply the paste to the red hive marks. As soon as the paste gets crumbly dry, apply more paste.

Add 1 cup of baking soda to a bath and soak in it for twenty minutes. Also, drink ¼ to ½ teaspoon of baking soda in a glass of water.

‡ HANDS—CHAPPED, ROUGH, AND RED

Chapped hands will be greatly soothed when you massage wheat germ oil into them.

Red, rough, and sore hands (feet, too) should be relieved with lemon juice. After you rinse off the lemon juice, massage the hands with olive, coconut, or wheat germ oil.

NOTE: Give a moisturizer time to work by keeping it on your hands overnight. To maximize the moisturizer's effectiveness, and to protect your linens, wear white cotton gloves to bed after you've put on the moisturizer. If you don't have white cotton gloves, then go to a photographic supply store and pick up the inexpensive gloves that photographers and film editors wear when handling film.

‡ CLEAN AND SOFTEN HANDS

In a jar, combine equal parts of tomato juice, lemon juice, and glycerin (available at drugstores). Let one hand massage the other with the mixture. Rinse with tepid water.

The ideal remedy for people with dry hands is their own sheep as a pet. Sheep's wool contains lanolin. By rubbing your hands across the animal's back every so often, you'll keep them in great shape.

‡ CHAPPED LIPS

Apply a thin film of glycerin (available at drugstores) to soften and protect your lips.

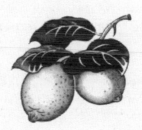

‡ BODY ODOR

"Think Zinc—Don't Stink!" Credit for that slogan goes to a Pennsylvania man who rid himself of body odor by taking 30 mg of zinc every day. Within two weeks, he was smelling like a rose.

Eat green leafy vegetables. They contain lots of chlorophyll. If your local health food store sells wheatgrass juice, buy and drink an ounce a day. Make sure you drink it on an empty stomach. All that chlorophyll should help combat body odor.

‡ SKUNK SPRAY

When you've gotten in the path of a frightened skunk, add a cup of tomato juice to a gallon of water and wash your body with it. Do the same with your clothes.

‡ SUMMER FRECKLES

Potato water (see "Preparation Guide") can help fade summer freckles. Dip a washcloth in it, wring it out, and apply it to the freckles. Leave it on for ten minutes daily. Incidentally, potato water is also good to use on frostbite. So, if you plan on staying outdoors for a long time—from summer to winter—make sure you have plenty of potatoes on hand . . . on foot . . . on face. . . .

Apply lemon juice, or juice of parsley, or juice of watercress.

If you get a whole lot of freckles, very close together, you'll have a nice suntan and won't have to bother with all this other stuff.

Combine 6 tablespoons of buttermilk with 1 teaspoon of grated horseradish. Since this is a mild skin bleach, coat the skin with a light oil before applying the mixture. Leave it on for twenty minutes, then wash it off with warm water. Follow up with a skin moisturizer on the bleached area.

For sensitive skin, apply some plain yogurt. Leave it on for fifteen minutes, then rinse off with cool water.

If you ever wake up in the morning, look in the mirror, and see freckles you never had before, try washing the mirror.

‡ STRETCH MARKS

After a shower or bath, gently massage sesame oil—about a tablespoon—all over your stretch-marked areas. Eventually, pregnancy and weight-loss stretch marks may disappear.

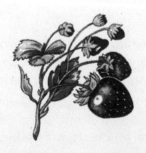

‡Sleep

Abraham Lincoln took a midnight walk to help him sleep. Charles Dickens believed it was impossible to sleep if you crossed the magnetic forces between the North and South Poles. As a result, whenever Mr. Dickens traveled, he took a compass with him so he could sleep with his head facing north.

Benjamin Franklin believed in fresh-air baths in the nude as a sleep inducer. During the night, he would move from one bed to another because he also thought that cold sheets had a therapeutic effect on him. (At least, that's what he told his wife!)

Mark Twain had a cure for insomnia: "Lie near the edge of the bed and you'll drop off."

According to Franklin P. Adams, "Insomniacs don't sleep because they worry about it and they worry about it because they don't sleep."

If you're caught up in this unhappy cycle of sleeplessness, try the suggestions on the next few pages.

‡ INSOMNIA

Exercise *during the day*. Get a real workout by taking a class or disciplining yourself at home by following a sensible exercise plan from a book or a videotape. DO NOT EXERCISE RIGHT BEFORE BEDTIME.

Try using an extra pillow. It works for some people.

Stay in one position. (Lying on the stomach is more relaxing than on the back.) Tossing and turning acts as a signal to the body that you're ready to get up.

In a pitch-black room, sit in a comfortable position with feet and hands uncrossed. Light a candle. Stare at the lit candle while relaxing each part of your body, starting with the toes and working your way up. Include ankles, calves, knees, thighs, genital area, stomach, waist, midriff, rib cage, chest, fingers, wrists, elbows, arms, shoulders, neck, jaw, lips, cheeks, eyes, eyebrows, forehead, and top of the head. Once your entire body is relaxed, blow out the candle and go to sleep.

Take your mind off *having* to fall asleep. Give yourself an interesting but unimportant fantasy type problem to solve. For instance: If you were to write your autobiography, what would be the title?

Steep 1 teaspoon of chamomile in a cup of boiling water for ten minutes and drink it right before bedtime.

Do not go to bed until you're really sleepy, even if it means going to bed very late when you have to get up early the next morning. Nothing will happen to you if you get less than eight, seven, six, or even five hours' sleep one night.

Get into bed. Before you lie down, breathe deeply six times. Count to 100, then breathe deeply another six times. Good night!

An hour before bedtime, peel and cut up a large onion. Pour 2 cups of boiling water over it and let it steep for fifteen minutes. Strain the water, then drink as much of it as you can. Do your evening ablutions (which might include freshening your breath), and go to sleep.

Folk-remedy recipes always include warm milk with ½ teaspoon of nutmeg and 1 or 2 teaspoons of honey before bedtime to promote restful sleep. The National Institute of Mental Health believes it works because warm milk contains tryptophan. Tryptophan is an essential amino acid or link of protein that increases the amount of serotonin in the brain. Serotonin is a neurotransmitter that helps to send messages from brain to nerves and vice versa. The advantage of a tryptophan-induced sleep over sleeping pills is that you awaken at the normal time every day and do not feel sleepy or drugged.

The feet seem to have a lot to do with a good night's sleep. One research book says, before going to bed, put the feet in the refrigerator for ten minutes. If you're brave (or silly) enough to try this, please proceed with care. Talk about getting cold feet . . .

Try a little Chinese acupressure. Press the center of the bottoms of your heels with your thumbs. Keep pressing as long as you can—at least three minutes. (Well, it beats sticking your feet in the fridge.)

If you've reached the point where you're willing to try just about anything, then rub the soles of your feet and the nape of your neck with a peeled clove of garlic. It may help you fall asleep.

Prevent sleepless nights by eating salt-free dinners and eliminating all after-dinner snacks. Try it a few nights in a row and see if it makes a difference in your night's sleep.

It is most advisable, for purposes of good digestion, not to have eaten two or three hours before bedtime. However, a remedy recommended by many cultures throughout the

CHICKEN SOUP & OTHER FOLK REMEDIES · 159

world as an effective cure for insomnia requires you to eat a finely chopped raw onion before going to bed.

Guilt-free masturbation is a wonderful relaxant and sleep inducer.

Totally satisfying sex is a great and fun sleep promoter. Unsatisfying sex can cause frustration that leads to insomnia. So (with apologies to Tennyson), is it better to have loved and lost sleep than never to have loved at all?

‡ NIGHTMARES

Right before going to sleep, soak your feet in warm water for ten minutes. Then rub them thoroughly with half a lemon. Don't rinse them off, just pat them dry. Take a few deep breaths and have pleasant dreams.

As you're dozing, tell yourself that you want to have happy dreams. It works lots of times.

This antinightmare advice comes from Switzerland: Eat a small evening meal about two hours before bedtime. When you go to bed, sleep on your right side with your right hand under your head.

Before you go to sleep, drink thyme tea and be nightmare-free.

Simmer the outside leaves of a head of lettuce in 2 cups of boiling water for fifteen minutes. Strain and drink the lettuce tea right before bedtime. It's supposed to ensure sweet dreams and is also good for cleansing the system.

‡ SNORING (POSSIBLE SLEEP APNEA)

A friend told us he starts to snore as soon as he falls asleep. We asked if it bothers his wife. He said, "It not only bothers my wife, it bothers the whole congregation."

Actually, *snoring* is not a joking matter. Chronic snoring, that is, snoring every night and loudly, may be the start of a serious condition known as sleep apnea. Apnea is Greek for "without breath." During the night, the windpipe keeps blocking the air as the throat relaxes and closes, making it difficult to breathe. After holding one's breath for an unnatural amount of time (anywhere from ten seconds to a couple of minutes), the snore comes as the person gasps for air. The person awakens each time it happens, and it can happen dozens and dozens of times during the night, without the person realizing it. The interrupted sleep causes that person to be tired all day. If you have this condition, it can be dangerous being behind the wheel of a car, operating heavy machinery, or just crossing a street. Aside from the daytime accident aspect, sleep apnea may lead to high blood pressure, heart problems, and stroke.

If you think that you may have sleep apnea, ask your doctor to recommend a sleep specialist right away. There are sleep clinics throughout the country.

Meanwhile, all snorers can minimize or completely eliminate their nighttime noise three ways:

- If you smoke, stop! Let your smoker's inflamed, swollen throat tissues heal.
- If you drink, don't! Alcoholic beverages relax the respiratory system muscles, making it harder to breathe and, in turn, promoting snoring.
- If you're overweight, trim down! Fat deposits at the base of the tongue contribute to the blocking of an already-clogged airway. Also, wait a couple of hours af-

ter you've eaten before going to sleep, and eating anything that will create additional congestion.

You may want to try sewing a tennis ball on the back of
the snorer's pajama top or nightgown. This prevents the
snorer from sleeping on his or her back, which prevents
snoring.

Snoring can be caused by very dry air—a lack of humidity
in the bedroom. If you use a radiator in cold weather, place
a pan of water on it, or simply use a humidifier.

‡Sore Throats

The trouble with sore throats is that each swallow is a painful reminder that you have a sore throat.

Many sore throats are caused by a mild viral infection that attacks when your resistance is low.

If you have a sore throat right now, think about your schedule. Chances are, you've been pushing yourself like crazy, running around and keeping later hours than usual.

If you take it easy, get a lot of rest, flush your system by drinking nondairy liquids, and stay away from "heavy" foods, the remedies we suggest will be much more effective.

NOTE: Chronic or persistent sore throat pain should be checked by your health professional.

‡ SORE THROATS IN GENERAL

Add 2 teaspoons of apple cider vinegar to a cup of warm water.

DOSE: Gargle a mouthful, spit it out, then swallow a mouthful. Gargle a mouthful, spit it out, then swallow a mouthful. Keep this up till the liquid is all gone. An hour later, start all over.

Mix 1 teaspoon of cream of tartar with ½ cup of pineapple juice and drink it.

DOSE: Repeat every half hour until there's a marked improvement.

A singer we know says this works for her every time: Steep 3 nonherbal tea bags in a cup of just-boiled water. Leave them there until the water is as dark as it can get—almost black.

DOSE: While the water is still quite hot but bearable, gargle with the tea. DO NOT SWALLOW ANY OF IT. No one needs all that caffeine. Repeat every hour until you feel relief.

Warm ½ cup of coarse (kosher) salt in a frying pan. Then pour the warm salt in a large, clean, white handkerchief and fold it over and over so that none of the salt can ooze out. Wrap the salted hanky around the neck and wear it that way for an hour.

This was one of our great-aunt's favorite remedies. The only problem was she would get laryngitis explaining to everyone why she was wearing that salty poultice around her neck.

Next time you wake up with that sore throat feeling, add 1 teaspoon of sage to 1 cup boiling water. Steep for three to five minutes and strain.

DOSE: Gargle in the morning and at bedtime. It would be wise to swallow the sage tea.

Relief from a sore throat can come by inhaling the steam of hot vinegar. Take special care while inhaling vinegar vapors or any other kind for that matter. You don't have to get too close to the source of the steam for it to be effective.

Grate 1 teaspoon of horseradish and 1 piece of lemon peel. To that, add ⅛ teaspoon of cayenne pepper and 2 tablespoons of honey.

DOSE: 1 tablespoon every hour.

We came across a beneficial exercise to do when you have a sore throat. Stick out the tongue for thirty seconds, put it back in and relax for a couple of seconds, then stick out the tongue again for another thirty seconds. Do it five times in a row and it will increase blood circulation, help the healing process, and make you the center of attention at the next executive board meeting.

What's a sore throat without honey and lemon? Every family has their own variation on the combination. Take the juice of a nice lemon (our family prefaces every noun with the word *nice*) and mix it with 1 teaspoon of some nice honey.

DOSE: Take it every two hours.

OR

Add the juice from 1 lemon to a glass of hot water (our family drinks everything from a glass) and sweeten to taste with honey—about 1½ tablespoons.

DOSE: 1 glass every four hours.

‡ HOARSENESS/LARYNGITIS

The trouble with laryngitis is that you have to wait until you don't have it before you can tell anyone you have it.

Rest your vocal cords as much as possible. If you have to talk, talk in a normal voice, letting the sound come from your diaphragm instead of your throat. DON'T WHISPER! Whispering tightens the muscles of your voice box, and puts more stress on your vocal cords than does talking in your normal voice.

Drink a mixture of 2 teaspoons of onion juice to 1 teaspoon of honey.

DOSE: Those 3 teaspoons every three hours.

Drink a cup of hot peppermint tea with a teaspoon of honey. After a hard day at the office, it's very relaxing for the entire body as well as the throat.

In 1 cup of water, simmer ½ cup of raisins for twenty minutes. Let it cool, then eat it all. This is a Tibetan remedy. It must work. We've never met anyone from Tibet with laryngitis.

Boil 1 pound of black beans in 1 gallon of water for one hour. Strain.

DOSE: 6 ounces of bean water an hour before each meal. The beans can be eaten during mealtime. (If necessary, see "Flatulence.")

When you're hoarse and hungry, eat baked apples. To prepare them, core 4 apples and peel them about halfway down from the top. Place them in a greased dish with about ½ inch of water. Drop a teaspoon of raisins into each apple core, then drizzle a teaspoon of honey into each core and over the tops of the apples. Cover and bake in a 350-degree oven for forty minutes. Baste a few times during the forty minutes with pan juices.

DOSE: Eat it warm or at room temperature. An apple a day . . . you know the rest.

‡ THROAT TICKLE

Chew a couple of whole cloves to relieve throat tickle.

Eat a piece of well-done toast (preferably whole wheat).

‡ SCALDED THROAT

Two teaspoons of olive oil will soothe and coat the throat.

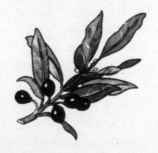

‡Stings and Bites

IF YOU HAVE A HISTORY OF AN ALLERGY TO STING-
ING INSECTS, HAVE A PHYSICIAN-PRESCRIBED EMER-
GENCY STING KIT ON HAND AT ALL TIMES!

This chapter deals with stings and bites from bees, wasps,
hornets, yellow jackets, mosquitoes, spiders, jellyfish, Por-
tuguese man-of-wars, hairy caterpillars, dogs, and snakes.

Everyone knows: to avoid disease from biting insects and
animals, don't bite any insects or animals! Should *they* bite
you, read on for practical and effective suggestions.

‡ BEE, WASP, HORNET, AND YELLOW JACKET STINGS

When an insect stings, its stinger usually remains in the
skin while the insect flies away. However, if the insect stays
attached to its stinger in the skin, flick it off with the
thumb and forefinger. DO NOT SQUEEZE THE INSECT, not
that anyone would want to do that.

Now then, remove the stinger, but do not use your fingers or tweezers. Those methods can pump more poison
into the skin. Instead, gently and carefully scrape the
stinger out with the tip of a sharp knife.

If you're into the dramatic, once the stinger is removed, suck the stung area like they do in snakebite-in-
the-desert movies. Spit out whatever poison comes out.
Every little bit of venom extracted will help minimize the
swelling.

To relieve the pain and keep down the swelling of a sting,
apply any one of the following for a half hour, then alternate it with a half hour of ice on the stung area:

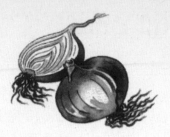

- A slice of raw onion
- A slice of raw potato
- Grated or sliced horseradish root
- Wet salt
- Commercial toothpaste
- Wet mud is one of the oldest and most practical remedies for stings. If you haven't already removed the stinger, peeling off the dry mud will help draw it out.
- Vinegar and lemon juice—equal parts—dabbed on every five minutes until the pain disappears.
- Watered-down ammonia
- ⅓ teaspoon of (unseasoned) meat tenderizer dissolved in 1 teaspoon of water. One of the main ingredients in meat tenderizer is papain, an enzyme from papaya that relieves the pain and inflammation of a sting as well as lessens allergic reaction. Use meat tenderizer only if you are MSG-allergy-free.
- Oil squeezed from a vitamin E capsule
- Wet a clump of tobacco and apply it to the sting, but don't tell the surgeon general or you'll have to print a warning on your arm.
- A drop of honey, preferably honey from the hive of the bee that did the stinging. (That's not too likely unless you're a beekeeper.)
- Apply a little of your own fresh urine. (It's great for unprepared campers.)

‡ JELLYFISH, PORTUGUESE MAN-OF-WAR, AND HAIRY CATERPILLAR STINGS

If you are stung by any of the above, immediately apply olive oil for fast relief, then seek medical attention.

‡ MOSQUITO BITES

Mosquitoes prefer warm over cold, light over dark, dirty over clean, adult over child, and male over female.

Once the mosquito bites the hand that feeds it, treat the bite with saliva. Then apply any of the following:

- Wet soap
- Wet tobacco
- Wet mud
- Watered-down ammonia
- Mixture of equal parts vinegar and lemon juice

As for the mosquito, after it bites you on one hand, give it the other hand, palm downward!

‡ SPIDER BITES

Four types of spiders have bites that can be serious:

- The black widow spider has a black shiny body and a red or orange hourglass marking on the underside of its abdomen.
- The brown recluse spider is also called the fiddle-back spider because of the violin-shaped marking on its back. It's found mainly in Southern and Midwestern states.
- The hobo spider is brown with a herringbone-like pattern on the top of its abdomen. It's found in the Pacific Northwest.

• The yellow sac spider is light yellow with a slightly darker stripe on the upper middle of its abdomen.

If you think the spider that bit you is any one of the above, try to remain as calm as possible and call your doctor, a hospital, and/or the Poison Information Center. If you can collect the spider, or any part of it, do so for identification purposes.

Until you get professional help, apply ice on the bite to help prevent swelling. A poultice of raw, grated potato on the bite would also be good.

Take nutrients that have anti-inflammatory action: vitamin C with bioflavonoids, 500 to 1000 mgs every two hours for several days (cut back on the dosage if you get diarrhea); bromelain, 500 mgs three or four times a day on an empty stomach; and/or quercetin, 250 to 300 mgs one to three times a day.

‡ ANIMAL BITES

An animal bite, even from your own pet dog, cat, hamster, guinea pig, ferret, or parakeet, could be dangerous. If the bite breaks the skin, bacteria in their saliva can cause infection.

Wash the bitten area thoroughly with soap and water. Apply pressure to stop the bleeding. Cover it loosely with a sterile bandage. If it doesn't stop bleeding, or if it puffs up, or is red and painful, see a doctor. You may need a tetanus shot.

If you're bitten by a wild animal—a dog, squirrel, or other rodent—see a doctor immediately. You may need a rabies vaccine.

‡ SNAKEBITES

If you get a snakebite, chances are you're expecting you might get a snakebite. Think that over for a minute. As soon as it makes sense, please read on. If you're going camping, or are placing yourself in a situation where there's a chance of being bitten by a snake, we recommend that you know the snakes in your area and keep an appropriate snakebite kit handy. If you do get bitten, and you've just run out of snakebite kit, make a poultice out of 2 crushed onions mixed with a few drops of kerosene and apply it to the bite. After a short time, it should draw out the poison, turning the poultice green. Or, do *you* turn green and the poultice . . . never mind. If you're near civilization, forget the above and get to a doctor!

Mix a wad of tobacco with saliva or water. Apply this paste directly on the bite. As soon as the paste dries, replace it with another wad of the paste and get to a doctor!

‡ RATTLESNAKE BITES

Don't get rattled. Wet some salt, put a hunk of it on the bite, then wrap the area with a wet-salt poultice. Don't stand around reading this. GET TO A DOCTOR!

‡Teeth, Gums, and Mouth

BE TRUE TO YOUR TEETH, OR THEY WILL BE FALSE TO YOU!

George Bernard Shaw said, "The man with toothache thinks everyone happy whose teeth are sound."

Home remedies can help ease the pain of a toothache and, in some cases, alleviate teeth problems caused by nervous tension and low-grade infections.

Since it is difficult to know what is causing the toothaches, make an appointment to see your dentist as soon as possible. More important, have the dentist see you.

‡ TOOTHACHE

When the pain of a toothache is driving you to extraction, here's how you can get relief until you get to the dentist:

Grate horseradish root and place a poultice of it behind the ear closest to the aching tooth. To ensure relief, also apply some of the grated horseradish to the gum area closest to the aching tooth.

Pack powdered milk in a painful cavity for temporary relief.

Acupressure works like magic for some people; hopefully you are one of them. If your toothache is on the right side, squeeze the index finger on your right hand (the one next to your thumb), on each side of your fingernail. As you're squeezing your finger, rotate it clockwise, giving that index finger a rapid little massage.

Apply just a few grains of cayenne pepper to the affected tooth and gum. At first it will add to the pain, but as soon as the smarting stops (within seconds), so should the toothache.

Soak a cheek-size piece of brown paper bag in vinegar, then sprinkle one side with black pepper. Place the peppered side on the side of the face with the toothache. Secure it in place with an Ace bandage and keep it there at least an hour.

Split open 1 fresh, ripe fig. Squeeze out the juice of the fruit onto your aching tooth. Put more fig juice on the tooth in fifteen-minute intervals, until the pain stops, or until you run out of fig juice. This is an ancient Hindu remedy. It must really work. When was the last time you saw an ancient Hindu with a toothache?

Roast ½ onion. Then, while it's still hot, place it on the pulse of your wrist on the opposite side of your troublesome tooth. By the time the onion cools completely, the pain should be gone.

An old standard painkiller is cloves. You can buy oil of cloves or whole cloves. The oil should be soaked in a wad of cotton and placed directly on the aching tooth. The whole clove should be dipped in honey that's been heated. Then, chew the clove slowly, rolling it around the aching tooth. That will release the essential oil and ease the pain.

Saturate a slice of toast with alcohol, then sprinkle on some pepper. The peppered side should be applied externally to the toothache side of the face.

If you love garlic, this one's for you. Place 1 just-peeled clove of garlic directly on the aching tooth. Keep it there for a minimum of one hour. ("Bad Breath" remedies soon follow.)

‡ TOOTH EXTRACTIONS

TO STOP BLEEDING: Dip a tea bag in boiling water, squeeze out the water, and allow it to cool. Then, pack the tea bag down on the tooth socket and keep it there for fifteen to thirty minutes.

TO STOP PAIN: Mix 1 teaspoon of Epsom salts with 1 cup of hot water. Swish the mixture around in your mouth and spit it out. DO NOT SWALLOW IT UNLESS YOU NEED A LAXATIVE. One cup should do the trick. If the pain recurs, get the Epsom salts and start swishing again.

Wrap an ice cube in gauze or cheesecloth. Hopefully you'll figure this out before the ice melts. When your thumb is up against the index finger, a meaty little tuft is formed where the fingers are joined. Acupuncturists call it the "hoku point." Spread your fingers and, with the ice cube, massage that tuft for seven minutes. If your hand starts to feel numb, stop massaging with the ice and continue with just a finger massage. It should give you from fifteen to thirty minutes of "no pain." This is also effective when you have pain after root canal work.

‡ LOOSE TEETH

Strengthen your teeth with parsley. Pour 1 quart of boiling water over 1 cup of parsley. Let it stand for fifteen minutes, then strain and refrigerate the parsley water.

DOSE: Drink 3 cups a day.

‡ PLAQUE REMOVER

Dampen your dental floss and dip it in baking soda, then floss with it. It may help remove some of the plaque buildup.

‡ GUMS (PYORRHEA AND GINGIVITIS)

Brian R. Clement, director of the Hippocrates Health Institute in West Palm Beach, Florida, reports that garlic is the first and foremost remedy for clearing up gum problems. He also warns that raw garlic can also burn sensitive gums. It is for that reason the Institute's professional staff mixes pectin with garlic before impacting the gums with it. The garlic heals the infection while the pectin keeps it from burning the gums. Suggest this line of defense to a (new age or holistic) periodontist.

Take Coenzyme Q-10—15 mg—twice a day. Also, open a Co-Q-10 capsule and use the powder in it for brushing your teeth and massaging your gums.

Each time you take a Co-Q-10, also take 500 mg of vitamin C with bioflavonoids.

‡ BLEEDING GUMS

Bleeding gums may be your body's way of saying you do not have a well-balanced diet. After checking with your dentist, you might consider seeking professional help from a vitamin therapist or nutritionist, to help you supplement your food intake with the vitamins and minerals you're lacking. Meanwhile, take 500 mg of vitamin C twice a day.

NOTE: Persistent bleeding gums should be investigated by a health professional.

‡ CARE AND CLEANING OF TEETH AND GUMS

Cut 1 fresh strawberry in half and rub your teeth and gums with it. It may help remove stains, discoloration, and tartar without harming the enamel. It may also strengthen and heal sore gums. Leave the crushed strawberry and juice on the teeth and gums as long as possible—at least fifteen minutes. Then rinse with warm water. USE FRESH STRAWBERRIES ONLY, AND AT ROOM TEMPERATURE.

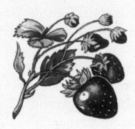

Actually, the proper way to clean your teeth is the way you do it right before leaving for your dental appointment.

If you can't brush after every meal, kiss someone. Really, kiss someone. It starts the saliva flowing and helps prevent tooth decay.

‡ BAD BREATH (HALITOSIS)

Stand in front of a mirror and stick out your tongue. Does it look coated, particularly the back half? If it is coated, you need to brush it just as you brush your teeth. A brushed tongue can eliminate bad breath, so go to it. You may want to buy a tongue scraper at the drugstore.

‡ GARLIC OR ONION BREATH

Mix ½ teaspoon of baking soda into a cup of water, then swish it, one gulp at a time, around your mouth. Spit out; do not swallow this mouthwash. By the time you've rinsed with the entire cup, your breath should be fresh.

Chew sprigs of parsley, yes, especially after eating garlic. Take your choice: garlic breath or little pieces of green stuff between your teeth.

If you're a coffee drinker, drink a strong cup of coffee to remove all traces of onion from your breath. Of course, then you have coffee breath, which, to some people, is just as objectionable as onion breath. Eat an apple. That will get rid of the coffee breath. In fact, forget the coffee and just eat an apple.

Chew a clove to sweeten your breath. People have been doing that for over five thousand years.

‡ MOUTHWASH

Prepare your own mouthwash by combining ¼ cup of apple cider vinegar with 2 cups of just-boiled water. Let it cool and store it in a jar in your medicine cabinet. Swish a mouthful of this antiseptic solution as you would with commercial mouthwash, for about one minute, and spit out. Then, be sure to rinse with water to remove the acid statis.

‡ DRYNESS OF MOUTH

Mix 1 tablespoon of honey with ½ cup of warm water and swish and gargle with it for about three to five minutes. Then rinse away the sweetness with water. The levulose in honey increases the secretion of saliva, relieving dryness of the mouth and making it easier to swallow.

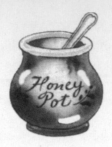

‡ CANKER SORES

Yogurt with active cultures (make sure the container specifies living or active cultures) may ease the condition faster than you can say *Lactobacillus acidophilus*. In fact, lactobacillus tablets may be an effective treatment for canker sores. Again, make sure the tablets have living organisms. Start by taking 2 tablets at each meal, then decrease the dosage as the condition clears.

Until you get to a health food store for the *Lactobacillus acidophilus*, dip 1 regular (nonherbal) tea bag in boiling water. Squeeze out most of the water. When it's cool to the touch, apply it to the canker sore for three minutes.

Take a mouthful of sauerkraut juice (use fresh from the barrel or in a jar found at health food stores, rather than the cans found in supermarkets) and swish it over the canker sore for about a minute. Then either swallow the juice or spit it out. Do this throughout the day, four to six times, every day until the sore is gone. It may disappear in only a day or two. If you're like me, you'll come to love the juice. You may even want to make your own sauerkraut. (See "Preparation Guide.")

‡ COLD SORES

The second a cold sore is on its way, there's a peculiar tingling sensation. At the first sign of that tingle, take *colorless* nail polish and paint it lightly on the area where the cold sore is about to emerge. The nail polish prevents the sore from blossoming. Television producer Cyndi Antoniak got this unique remedy from her dermatologist. Since Cyndi first used this remedy successfully some time ago, she's not had to use it again. Incidentally, the polish peels off naturally within a short time.

‡Urinary Problems

The urinary system includes the kidneys, ureters, bladder, and urethra.

Many of the remedies are helpful for more than one condition. Therefore, most of the bladder and kidney ailments (infections, stones, inflammation, etc.) are bunched together under "Urinary Problems."

We suggest you read them all in order to determine the most appropriate one(s) for your specific problem.

‡ URINARY PROBLEMS IN GENERAL

Urinary infections, kidney stones, gravel, and inflammation of the bladder and kidneys should all be evaluated by a health professional. Along with his or her recommendations are the following worth-a-try remedies that may ease your condition:

Drink plenty of fluids, including parsley tea—3 to 4 cups a day. If you have a juicer, 1 or 2 glasses of parsley juice, daily, should prove quite beneficial. Also, sprinkle fresh parsley on the foods you eat. You may start to see improvements any time from three days to three weeks.

Onions are a diuretic and will help to cleanse your system. Also, for kidney stimulation, apply a poultice of grated or finely chopped onions to the kidney area—the small of the back.

Pure cranberry juice (no sugar or preservatives added) has been known to help heal kidney and bladder infections.
DOSE: 6 ounces of room-temperature cranberry juice three times a day.

Carrot tops and celery tops are tops in strengthening the kidneys and bladder. In the morning, cover a bunch of scrubbed carrot tops with 12 ounces of boiled water and let them steep. Drink 4 ounces of the carrot-top water before each meal. After each meal, eat a handful of scrubbed celery tops. Within five weeks, there should be a noticeable and positive difference in the kidneys and bladder.

Pumpkin seeds are high in zinc and good for strengthening the bladder muscle.
DOSE: 1 palmful of unprocessed (unsalted) shelled pumpkin seeds three times a day.

According to the American Indians, corn silk (the silky strands beneath the husk of corn) is a cure-all for urinary problems. The most desirable corn silk is from young corns, gathered before the silk turns brown. Take a handful of corn silk and steep it in 3 cups of boiled water for five minutes. Strain and drink the 3 cups throughout the day. Corn silk can be stored in a glass jar, not refrigerated. If you can't get corn silk, use corn silk extract, available at most health food stores. Add 10 to 15 drops of the extract to a cup of water.

According to a book, *The Elements of Materia Medica,* edited in 1854, asparagus was a popular remedy for kidney stones. It is said that asparagus acts to increase cellular activity in the kidneys and helps break up oxalic acid crystals.

DOSE: A half cup of cooked and blended or puréed asparagus before breakfast and before dinner, or boil 1 cup of asparagus in 2 quarts of water and drink a cup of the asparagus water four times a day.

After eating asparagus, you may notice that your urine has an unusual smell. There are a few scientific theories as to what causes that specific smell. In 1891, the experiments of a researcher named Nencki led him to conclude that the scent is due to a metabolite called *methanethiol*. This odoriferous chemical is said to be produced as your body metabolizes asparagus. Some say that the smell is a sign of kidney-bladder cleansing; others believe it indicates faulty secretion of gastric hydrochloric acid (HCL).

A respected French herbalist recommends eating almost nothing but strawberries for three to five days, for relief of kidney stones. ANY FAST OR DRAMATIC CHANGE OF DIET SHOULD BE SUPERVISED BY A HEALTH PROFESSIONAL!

‡ INCONTINENCE
Incontinence should be evaluated by a health professional. In addition, you might try directing the stream of water from an ordinary garden hose to the soles of the feet for up to two minutes. It has been known to reduce incontinence, particularly in older people. It also helps circulation in the feet.

‡ DIURETICS
To stimulate urination try any of the following in moderation, using good common sense by listening to your body:

• Celery: cooked in chicken soup or raw in salads
• Watercress: soup or salads
• Leek: mild diuretic in soup, much stronger when eaten raw, and a perfect basis for a cheap joke about urination

- Parsley: in soup, salads, juiced, or as a tea
- Asparagus: raw or cooked and as a tea
- Cucumber: raw
- Corn silk: tea
- Onions: raw in salads and/or rub your loins with sliced onions (Yes. You read that correctly.)
- Horseradish: Grate ½ cup of horseradish and boil it with ½ cup of beer. Drink this concoction three times a day.
- Watermelon: Eat a piece first thing in the morning and do not eat other foods for at least two hours.

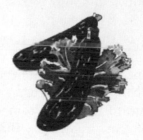

‡ VERY FREQUENT URINATION

Cherry juice or cranberry juice (no sugar or preservatives added) has been said to help regulate the problem of constantly having to urinate.

DOSE: Drink 3 to 4 glasses of cherry or cranberry juice throughout the day. Be sure it's room temperature, not chilled.

NOTE: Persistent frequent urination may be a sign of a urinary tract infection or diabetes and should be checked by a health professional.

‡ BEDWETTING

See "Infants and Children."

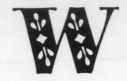

‡Warts

‡ WARTS IN GENERAL

No matter how you feel about warts, they have a way of growing on you.

Verruca vulgaris is the medical term for the common wart. (Don't you think a wart looks like a *Verruca vulgaris*?)

Warts usually appear on the hands, feet, and face, and are believed to be caused by a virus.

The "quantity" award for home remedies goes to warts. We got a million of 'em—remedies, that is, not warts.

We tried to get warts for research purposes. We kept touching frogs. It's a fallacy. You do not get warts from touching frogs. (Incidentally, you do not get a prince from kissing them either.)

If you have a wart, here are a wide variety of treatments from which to find the one that works for you.

Crush a fresh fig until it has a mushy consistency and put it on the wart for a half hour each day. Keep doing that until the wart disappears.

First thing each morning, dab spittle on the wart.

Warts on the genitals? Gently rub the inner side of pineapple skin on the affected parts. Repeat every morning and evening until the warts are gone, or the pineapple's gone, or the parts are gone.

Apply a used tea bag to the wart for fifteen minutes a day. Within a week to ten days you should be wartless.

Pick some dandelions. Break the stems and put the juice that oozes out of the stems directly on the wart—once in the morning and once in the evening, five days in a row.

If you have warts on your body, you may have too much lime in your system. One way to neutralize the excess lime is to drink a cup of chamomile tea two or three times a day.

Grate carrots and combine them with a teaspoon of olive oil. Put the mixture on the wart for a half hour twice a day.

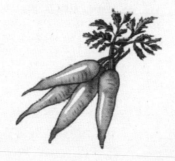

Dab lemon juice on the wart, immediately followed by a raw chopped onion. Do that twice a day, fifteen minutes each time.

Put a fresh slice of raw potato on the wart and keep it in place with a bandage. Leave it on overnight. Take it off in the morning. Then repeat the procedure again at night. If you don't get rid of the wart in a week, replace the potato with a clove of garlic.

Every morning, squish out the contents of a vitamin E capsule and rub it vigorously on the wart. This remedy is slow (more than a month) but what's the rush?

Dab on the healing juice of the aloe vera plant every day until the wart disappears.

If you don't have the patience to tend to the wart on a daily basis, consider finding a competent, professional hypnotist. Warts can actually be hypnotized away.

‡ PLANTAR WARTS

At bedtime, puncture 1 or 2 garlic pearles (soft gels) and squeeze out the oil on the plantar warts. Massage the oil on the entire area for a few minutes. Put a clean white sock on your foot and leave it on while you sleep. Do this every night for a week or two, until the little black roots come out and fall off.

‡Weight Control Tips

Whether you've spent years yo-yoing your way through one diet after another and are heavier than ever, or just need to lose a few pounds to look better in that bathing suit, here are suggestions to healthfully help you shed those unwanted pounds.

‡ SLOW AND STEADY WINS THE RACE

Change your lifestyle habits gradually. The key word is "gradually." *Gradually,* day by day, replace a couple of fattening foods with healthier choices. In doing so, you become super-aware of what you're eating. That's a major step in improving your daily food intake.

Also, *gradually* start exercising. Maybe walk briskly for ten minutes the first few days, then twelve minutes, then fifteen, and keep going until you work your way up to doing a supervised exercise program that's appropriate for you.

Be happy if you lose up to two pounds a week. In terms of keeping the weight off permanently, losing no more than two pounds a week makes sense. If you lose more, your body thinks you're going to starve, and, in an effort to protect you from dying of hunger, it will slow down your metabolism. A loss of one or two pounds a week adds up to a big difference in a matter of months. And that's weight that will most likely *stay off*.

‡ FOODS THAT ARE FILLING

Plan on eating foods that have a high water content. Prepare meals with fruits and vegetables—soups, stews, and smoothies. An apple is 84 percent water, amounting to almost 4 ounces of water. Broccoli, ½ cup, cooked, is 91 percent water, giving you 2.4 ounces of water. Look how much water it takes to make rice. (Spaghetti, too.) High-water-content foods will fill you up and hydrate you at the same time.

‡ SNACKS

Fruit is a great, easy-to-prepare, fibrous, health-giving, sweet treat. We could fill a book naming each fruit, its nutritional value, and ways to prepare it. Instead, we suggest that you be adventurous and creative. Go to your green-grocer or any ethnic market and find exotic fruit to add to your repertoire. Be sure to clean fruit before you eat them. (For a super cleaner, see "Healthful and Helpful Hints.")

Ever think of having a sweet potato or a yam as a snack? "Yam" comes from the Guinean word for "something to eat." It's something *wonderful* to eat! Yams are rich in potassium; sweet potatoes are rich in vitamin A; both are good sources of folate, the heart-protective vitamin B, and vitamin C. Both are easy to prepare, fat-free, and worth the 100 to 140 satisfying calories.

When you crave something crunchy, get out the finger vegetables. Chomp on baby carrots, jicama and fennel sticks, strips of yellow or red bell pepper, and the old standby, celery. On a weekend morning, prepare a bowl of the cut-up vegetables. Keep them in ice water in your refrigerator, and reach for it whenever you need to nibble.

‡ HIGH-PROTEIN LUNCH

If you have a high-protein lunch—fish, soy products, yogurt, meat, chicken—you may find yourself eating fewer calories for dinner. Protein—2 or 3 ounces—is said to trigger a hormone that cuts your appetite and leaves you feeling satisfied. Give it a try. Stay away from high-carbohydrate noon meals—pasta, rice, potatoes—and see if a portion of protein (along with veggies or salad—the good stuff) helps reduce your calorie intake at dinner.

‡ FAT'S WHERE IT'S AT

"An unlikely hero in the battle of the bulge is, in fact, classified as a fat," says Jade Beutler, licensed health care practitioner, author of *Understanding Fats and Oils, Your Guide to Healing with Essential Fatty Acids* and *Flax for Life*, and a foremost authority on the many benefits of flaxseed oil. According to Beutler's research findings, flaxseed oil can help:

- Decrease cravings for fatty foods and sweets
- Stoke metabolic rate
- Creates satiation (feeling of fullness and satisfaction following a meal)
- Regulate blood sugar
- Regulate insulin levels
- Increase oxygen consumption

The ideal method of taking flaxseed oil for purposes of weight loss or maintenance is 1 to 2 tablespoons daily, in divided doses taken with each meal.

Jade Beutler is affiliated with Barlean's Organic Oils. After doing our own flaxseed oil product research, we're now using Barlean's Lignan Rich Flax Oil. It's costly but we feel it's worth it. See more details about flaxseed oil in "And Now May We Prevent . . ." Before you do, check out "Cellulite Eliminator" (below) to read the testimony of a friend who volunteered her experience with flaxseeds.

‡ CELLULITE ELIMINATOR

Former model Maureen Klimt is getting older *and* better. Determined to get rid of cellulite, she started taking omega-3 fatty acids in the form of flaxseeds. Maureen grinds the seeds in a little coffee grinder, sprinkles 1 to 2 tablespoons on oatmeal, and then adds a touch of maple syrup. After eating the flaxseeded oatmeal daily for months, she reports the cellulite is no longer there. Although Maureen eats healthy and exercises, she credits the flaxseeds for the loss of cellulite.

‡ FIRM THIGHS

Sonoma Mission Inn Spa & Country Club is sharing their once-secret treatment for jiggly thighs. The key ingredient is rosemary. (No, that's *not* a physical trainer who gives you a workout.) Rosemary is an herb that stimulates circulation and drains impurities, leaving skin firmer and tighter. Mix 1 tablespoon of crushed dried rosemary (available at herb and health food stores) with 2 tablespoons of extra virgin olive oil. Smooth mixture over thighs; wrap in plastic wrap and leave on for ten minutes. Then rinse the mixture off your thighs. Do this treatment at least once a week.

‡ WAYS TO REV UP YOUR METABOLISM

Kelp is seaweed that's rich in minerals and vitamins, especially the B family. Its high iodine content helps activate a sluggish thyroid. Dried kelp can be eaten raw, or crumbled into soups and on salads. Powdered kelp can also be used in place of salt. It has a salty, fishy taste that may take getting used to. If you really don't like the taste, there are kelp pills. Follow the recommended dosage on the label. One of the good side effects of kelp is that it may make your hair shinier. If you eat too much kelp, it can have a laxative effect.

At England's Oxford Polytechnic Institute, a study showed that adding 1 teaspoon of hot-pepper sauce (something with cayenne pepper, like Tabasco Sauce) and 1 teaspoon of mustard to every meal raised one's metabolic rate by as much as 25 percent.

Before you eat dinner, exercise for twenty to thirty minutes. Just plain walking will do. Exercise boosts your metabolic rate and it lasts through dinner, helping you digest and burn off the evening meal. For many, that before-dinner walk seems to reduce the urge for late-night snacks.

Do not eat within three hours of going to sleep. The body seems to store fat more easily at night, when the metabolism slows down.

‡ WHY WATER OR JUICE

The impactful results of a study reported in the *American Journal of Clinical Nutrition* shows that drinking water or juice before a meal, rather than beer, wine, or a cocktail, goes a long way with weight control. The imbibers consumed an average of 240 calories in their alcoholic beverage, and wolfed down about 200 more calories in their meal. They also ate faster. It took them longer to feel full, but that didn't stop them. They continued eating past the point of feeling full. And all that because they had an alcoholic drink before their meal. Water, waiter, please!

‡ WHY NOT SODA

It's been reported that people who are frequent diet- or nondiet-soda drinkers have higher hunger ratings than people who drink unsweetened or naturally sweet beverages. Experiment by going off all soda for a week to see if your desire for food decreases.

‡ DOGGY BAGS

As soon as you're served food at a restaurant, ask for a doggy bag. Explain that you're into "portion control," and don't want to tempt yourself to finish everything on the plate.

‡ HOLIDAYS—THE TOUGH TIMES

Forget about losing weight during holidays. Settle for not *gaining* weight. Fill up on sweet potatoes, fruits, vegetables, white meat turkey, whole-grain bread, and an occasional tiny portion of an obscenely fattening dessert.

Eat healthy, nonfattening food right before you go to a holiday party.

At a holiday event, drink designer water, or sparkling water with a twist of lemon. A little wine is okay, but stay away from mixed drinks or liqueurs.

According to Alan Hirsch, M.D., director of the Smell & Taste Treatment and Research Foundation in Chicago, "People who are exposed to smells of food during the day eat less at night." Proof that this may be so is evident during Ramadan, the Muslim holiday of daytime fasting followed by nighttime feasting. Muslim women's hunger ratings dropped, but men's hunger stayed the same throughout the month-long holiday. Then again, the women prepared food all day, and by mealtime, their hunger had abated. The food wasn't as appealing to them.

‡ THE GREAT OUTDOORS

A day without sunshine is like a day without serotonin, a brain chemical that can allay hunger. Your body needs sunlight to make serotonin, so get out there every chance you get. While you're outdoors, may as well get a little exercise, too. Walk. Play. Skip. Enjoy yourself! And don't forget the sunscreen.

‡ MIRROR, MIRROR, ON THE KITCHEN WALL

Studies were done with over one thousand people divided into groups who ate in front of mirrors and those who ate without seeing themselves in mirrors. The people who watched themselves chow down ate considerably less fat than those who were mirrorless.

A mirror in your kitchen may be the reminder that you need each time you decide on something to eat.

‡ THIS MAY BE THE MOTIVATION YOU NEED: DETERMINING YOUR WEIGHT/HEALTH PROFILE

Body Mass Index (BMI) is one of the most accurate ways to determine when extra pounds translate into health risks. BMI is a measure that takes into account a person's weight and height to gauge total body fat in adults.

According to the federal government guidelines, the definition of a healthy weight is a BMI of 24 or less. A BMI of 25 to 29.9 is considered overweight. Individuals who fall into the BMI range of 25 to 34.9, and have a waist size of over forty inches for men and thirty-five inches for women, are considered to be at especially high risk for health problems.

BMI is reliable for most people between nineteen and seventy years of age except women who are pregnant or breast feeding, competitive athletes, body builders, and chronically ill patients.

To use the table below, find the appropriate height in the column on the left. Move across to a given weight. The number at the top of the column is the BMI for that height and weight. Pounds have been rounded off.

‡ BODY MASS INDEX CHART

Height (inches)	19	20	21	22	23	24	25	26	27	28	29	30	31	32	33	34	35
									Body Weight (pounds)								
58	91	96	100	105	110	115	119	124	129	134	138	143	148	153	158	162	167
59	94	99	104	109	114	119	124	128	133	138	143	148	153	158	163	168	173
60	97	102	107	112	118	123	128	133	138	143	148	153	158	163	168	174	179
61	100	106	111	116	122	127	132	137	143	148	153	158	164	169	174	180	185
62	104	109	115	120	126	131	136	142	147	153	158	164	169	175	180	186	191
63	107	113	118	124	130	135	141	146	152	158	163	169	175	180	186	191	197
64	110	116	122	128	134	140	145	151	157	163	169	174	180	186	192	197	204
65	114	120	126	132	138	144	150	156	162	168	174	180	186	192	198	204	210
66	118	124	130	136	142	148	155	161	167	173	179	186	192	198	204	210	216
67	121	127	134	140	146	153	159	166	172	178	185	191	198	204	211	217	223
68	125	131	138	144	151	158	164	171	177	184	190	197	203	210	216	223	230
69	128	135	142	149	155	162	169	176	182	189	196	203	209	216	223	230	236
70	132	139	146	153	160	167	174	181	188	195	202	209	216	222	229	236	243
71	136	143	150	157	165	172	179	186	193	200	208	215	222	229	236	243	250
72	140	147	154	162	169	177	184	191	199	206	213	221	228	235	242	250	258
73	144	151	159	166	174	182	189	197	204	212	219	227	235	242	250	257	265
74	148	155	163	171	179	186	194	202	210	218	225	233	241	249	256	264	272
75	152	160	168	176	184	192	200	208	216	224	232	240	248	256	264	272	279
76	156	164	172	180	189	197	205	213	221	230	238	246	254	263	271	279	287

SOURCE: National Heart, Lung, and Blood Institute

‡And Now May We Prevent . . .

When we were doing research for this book, we came across preventive measures as well as treatments.

While we can't offer a guarantee with each one, we do believe that these healthful hints may help to offset the onset of specific ailments.

‡ PREVENTION TO THE MAX WITH FLAX

A deficiency of omega-3 has been positively correlated with over sixty illnesses, including: arthritis, atherosclerosis, cancer, diabetes, hypertension (high blood pressure), immune disorders, menopausal discomfort, and stroke. And so adding omega-3 supplementation to your daily diet may go a long way in helping to prevent, improve, or reverse those unhealthy conditions. Flax oil, processed from flaxseed, contains the highest concentration of *essential* omega-3 of any other source on the planet.

Flaxseed contains phyto-nutrients called lignans. Lignans are reported to have the following attributes: antitumor properties; estrogen-mimicking effect without the risks associated with estrogen therapy; powerful antioxidant capabilities; antiviral properties; antibacterial properties; and antifungal properties. Studies suggest that lignans may help prevent many health challenges including breast and colon cancer, and can help lower cholesterol, regulate women's menstrual cycle, and reduce or eliminate menopause symptoms.

If you're thinking that flaxseed, in some form, should be part of your daily diet, we think it's a wise decision. To help you decide which form(s) to take, you should know that flaxseeds have hard outer shells. You can eat them *after* you've soaked a few tablespoons of the seeds overnight. The most popular way to eat flaxseeds is to grind them in a spice or coffee grinder and sprinkle a tablespoon of the ground meal on your cereal, or add it to a smoothie, or mix it into a portion of yogurt or cottage cheese. When baking, you can replace a few tablespoons of your regular flour with flax flour.

To make sure we get our daily dose of the omega-3 oils and lignans, we find it most convenient to take flax oil. The daily recommended dose is one tablespoon of flax oil per every one hundred pounds of body weight. We take a tablespoon of it either in a smoothie—it doesn't change the taste of the smoothie, it just keeps it from getting very aerated—or we mix flax oil in fat-free cottage cheese, or fat-free yogurt, along with a minced clove of garlic. It's good! We also use flax oil in a homemade salad dressing. There are lots of recipes, too, using flax oil. See the "Recommended Reading" chapter.

When we first started looking for flax oil, we went to the refrigerated section of our local health food store and found Barlean's Flax Oil. It had all of the qualities we were looking for: The label said, "Lignan Rich." Also, due to flaxseed oil's limited shelf life—it's an oil that can become rancid and should be kept refrigerated—we checked the "pressing date" and the "best before date," making sure it didn't exceed a four-month span.

We got in touch with Barlean's Organic Oils to learn about the company and the integrity of their products. We were so impressed that we're mentioning them here. Call their toll-free number, 1-800-445-3529, and ask them to send you "Flax Facts 2000." The booklet has valuable information about the benefits of flaxseed oil. There are also a few recipes included.

‡ ARTERIOSCLEROSIS (HARDENING OF THE ARTERIES)

According to French folklore, eating rye bread made with baker's yeast supposedly prevents hardening of the arteries.

It is reported that some Russians eat mature, raw potatoes at every meal to prevent arteriosclerosis.

Drinking a combination of apple cider boiled with garlic once a day is a Slavic folk remedy that may not prevent arteriosclerosis, but it certainly tastes like it should.

‡ ARTHRITIS

Edgar Cayce, renowned psychic, said in one of his readings, "Those who would take a peanut oil rub each week need never fear arthritis."

‡ BALDNESS

Mix 1 jigger of vodka with ½ teaspoon of cayenne pepper and rub it on the scalp. The blood supply feeds the hair. The pepper and vodka stimulates the blood supply. If this doesn't work, there is a plus side to baldness—it prevents dandruff.

‡ CANCER

According to psychic healer Edgar Cayce, eat 3 almonds each day and you never need fear certain kinds of cancer.

‡ COLDS/FLU

The natural sulfur in broccoli and parsley is supposed to help us resist colds. Eat broccoli and/or parsley once a day.

An apple a day . . . A university study showed that the students who ate apples regularly had fewer colds.

The second you've been exposed to someone with the flu, try taking cinnamon oil.

DOSE: 5 drops of cinnamon oil in a tablespoon of water, three times a day.

By drinking raw sauerkraut juice once a day, you should avoid getting the flu. (It's also a good way to avoid constipation.)

Move to the North Pole for the winter. None of the standard cold- and flu-causing microorganisms can survive there. The problem is, you might not be able to either.

‡ DRUNKENNESS

Before you have a drink, sprinkle nutmeg into a glass of milk and sip it slowly. It may help absorb and neutralize the effects of alcoholic beverages.

You might be able to avert drunkenness by eating a handful of raw almonds on an empty stomach.

Aristotle advised his followers to eat a big chunk of cabbage before imbibing. Cole slaw—cabbage and vinegar—is said to be an even more effective intoxication preventive.

The best way to hold your liquor is in the bottle it comes in! What may help you to do that is, when sober, look at a man or woman who is drunk.

‡ DYSENTERY

To help prevent bacterial dysentery, two weeks before you travel to a foreign country, eat a finely chopped raw onion in a cup of yogurt every day. Before you discard this preventive measure, try it. You may be surprised at how good it tastes. The yogurt somehow makes the onion taste sweet.

‡ FAINTING SPELLS

If you're prone to fainting spells—a case of the vapors, perhaps—keep pepper handy. Sniff a grain or two and sneeze. The sneeze stimulates the brain's blood vessels and may help prevent fainting. It's good to remember, since not many households have smelling salts, but just about all have black pepper.

‡ FALLING ASLEEP

You don't have to depend on caffeine for staying awake. Mix 1 teaspoon of cayenne pepper to 1 quart of juice—any kind of juice with no sugar or preservatives added. Throughout a long drive, or a night of cramming, as soon as you feel sleep overcoming you, take a cup of the cayenne-laced juice to keep awake and alert.

‡ GAS/FLATULENCE

Drink ginger tea after a heavy, gassy meal. Steep ¼ teaspoon of powdered ginger in a cup of hot water for five minutes, or let a few small pieces of fresh gingerroot steep, then drink the tea slowly.

To prevent beans from giving you gas, soak the dried beans overnight. Next morning, pour off the water. Add fresh water and an onion, and boil them. When it comes to a boil, pour off the water and throw away the onion.

Then, cook the beans the way you ordinarily cook them, only this time, they may not create gas.

‡ GRAYING HAIR

According to the Chinese, a combination of fresh ginger-root juice and ground cloves should be massaged into the scalp to prevent gray hair.

‡ HANGOVERS

If you insist on drinking, you may be interested to know that a research team from England advises drinkers to guzzle clear alcohols—gin, vodka, or white rum—to lessen the chances of that "morning after" feeling. Red wine and whiskey seem to have more hangover-promoting elements.

‡ HAY FEVER

Find the nearest beekeeper in your vicinity and ask for honeycomb. Take a 1-inch square of it twice a day. Swallow the honey and chew the beeswax. After five or ten minutes, spit out the wax. Start this regime two months before hay fever time. By the time hay fever season rolls around, the honeycomb may have helped you build an immunity to the pollen in your area. If you don't have a local beekeeper, check out the honeycomb in your local health food store. Hopefully it's from your neck of the woods.

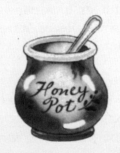

‡ HEART ATTACK

A cup of peppermint tea a day is said to help prevent a heart attack.

‡ HEMORRHOIDS

To prevent hemorrhoids, it's best to increase the fiber and fluids in your diet.

According to psychic healer Edgar Cayce, 3 raw almonds a day will not only help prevent cancer, they will help prevent hemorrhoids, too.

Since hemorrhoids are a sitter's ailment, it may help to take a long walk every day at a fairly fast pace. A yoga exercise class two or three times a week is also a good preventive measure.

‡ INDIGESTION

Add 1 cup of bran and 1 cup of oatmeal to a gallon of water. Let it stand for twenty-four hours, then strain, keeping the liquid. Drink a cup of it fifteen minutes before each meal to prevent indigestion.

To prevent indigestion by aiding digestion, see if this helps: Try not to drink any beverages during or after meals. Wait *at least* one hour, preferably two or three hours after eating, before drinking any liquids.

‡ INFECTIONS

According to a doctor quoted in a Roman newspaper, "Kissing is good for your health and will make you live longer." The doctor explains, "Kissing stimulates the heart, which gives more oxygen to the body's cells, keeping the cells young and vibrant." He also found that kissing produces antibodies in the human body that, in the long run, can protect the body against certain infections. (We wonder if his report was S.W.A.K.)

‡ INSECT BITES

If you are going into an area overrun with mosquitoes, and you know about it days in advance, take 100 mg of vitamin B_1 (thiamine) every day for a week before you leave for that infested area. Also take a B_1 an hour before you reach that spot.

Eucalyptus oil will repel mosquitoes. Rub it over the uncovered areas of your body.

Don't wear the color blue around mosquitoes. They're very attracted to it. They're also attracted to wet clothes. Keep dry!

Rub fresh parsley on the exposed parts of your body to prevent insect bites.

If you have an aloe vera plant, break off one of the stems. Squeeze out the juice and rub it on the uncovered areas of your body for protection against biting insects.

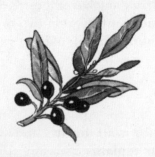

‡ KIDNEY STONES

A high level of oxalate in the urine contributes to the formation of most (calcium) kidney stones. If this problem runs in your family, or if you've already gone through the agony of a kidney stone, chances are you'll need to take every precaution to help prevent it from happening to you once or again. Completely eliminate, or at least limit, your intake of the foods and beverages that are high in oxalates or that can produce oxalic acid. That includes: caffeine—coffee, black tea (including orange pekoe), cocoa, chocolate—spinach, sorrel, asparagus, beets, Swiss chard, parsley, dried figs, poppy seeds, rhubarb, lamb's-quarters, purslane, nuts, and pepper.

Eat foods rich in vitamin A, the vitamin that can help discourage the formation of stones. They include: apricots, pumpkin, sweet potatoes, squash, carrots, and cantaloupe.

Start your day by drinking a glass of (distilled) water in which you squeezed the juice of a lemon. The citric acid and magnesium in the lemon may also help prevent the formation of kidney stones.

Most important is that you drink a lot of *good* water daily. Distilled water is ideal.

‡ MOTION SICKNESS

A Mexican method of preventing motion sickness is to keep a copper penny in the navel. It is supposed to work especially well on crowded bus rides over bumpy roads.

For at least half a day before leaving on a trip, have only liquid foods that are practically sugar-free and salt-free.

Pull out and pinch the skin in the middle of your inner wrist, about an inch from your palm. Keep pulling and pinching alternate wrists to prevent motion sickness. We advise you *not* to do this if you're doing the driving.

‡ NAUSEA

A cup of warm water one half hour before each meal may prevent nausea.

‡ NOSEBLEED

Help prevent nosebleeds by eating an orange a day. Be sure to eat the pith (that's the spongy white part that is loaded with bioflavonoids). This information came from the Linus Pauling Institute.

‡ PYORRHEA

Make your own toothpaste by combining baking soda with a drop or two of hydrogen peroxide. Brush your teeth and massage your gums with it, using a soft, thin-bristled brush.

NOTE: Pyorrhea or swollen gums should be evaluated by a dentist.

Take Coenzyme Q-10—15 mg—twice a day. Also, open a Co-Q-10 capsule and use the powder in it for brushing your teeth and massaging your gums.

Each time you take a Co-Q-10, also take 500 mg of vitamin C with bioflavonoids.

‡ SCIATICA

According to the Germans, eating a portion of raw sauerkraut every day prevents sciatica.

‡ SKIN CANCER

Before basking in the sun, you know, of course, to use a sunscreen with an SPF of 15 or more. But do you know that eating foods high in carotene—carrots, dandelion greens, watercress, kale, and sweet potatoes—might reduce the risk of skin cancer?

‡ SMOKING

If you want to stop or, at least, cut down on your cigarette or cigar smoking, after your next cigarette, replace the nicotine taste in your mouth by sucking on a small clove. An hour or two later, replace the clove with another one. Without that lingering nicotine taste, your desire for another cigarette should be greatly reduced.

‡ SNEEZING

If you feel a sneeze coming on and you're in a situation where a sneeze would be quite disruptive, put your finger on the tip of your nose and press in.

‡ STROKE

A cup of peppermint tea daily is said to reduce the chances of a stroke by 40 percent. The peppermint tea is rich in potassium, having several times the amount found in an average banana. If you're taking medication to help prevent a stroke, you'll want to read ANTICLOTTING MEDICATION ALERT on page 106.

‡ TOOTH PAIN

If you are scheduled to go to the dentist for work on your sensitive teeth, take 10 mg of vitamin B_1 every day, starting a week before your dental appointment. You may find that the pain during and after dental procedures will be greatly reduced. Vitamin B_1 is thiamine. It is thought that the body's lack of thiamine might be what lets the pain become severe in the first place.

‡ WRINKLES

Apply a facial made with equal parts of brewer's yeast and yogurt. When it dries on the skin, gently wash it off with warm water and pat dry. Give yourself a facial twice a week to help prevent wrinkles.

Buttermilk is a good wrinkle-preventing facial. Keep it on for about twenty minutes, then splash it off with warm water and pat dry.

This is supposedly the secret formula of a renowned French beauty: combine and boil 1 cup of milk, 2 teaspoons of lemon juice, and 1 tablespoon of brandy. While the mixture is warm, paint it on the face and neck with a pastry brush. When it is thoroughly dry, wash it off with warm water and pat dry.

Avoid excessive sun exposure.

‡Healthful and Helpful Hints

‡ NATURAL INSECT REPELLENTS

Ants steer clear of garlic. Rub a peeled clove of garlic on problem areas and they will be ant-free in no time.

Make pomanders using oranges and cloves (see "Preparation Guide"). Put a pomander in each clothes closet and say bye-bye to moths.

Flies are repelled by thyme tea. Fill a plant mister with a cup of thyme tea and spray around doors and windows to keep flies away.

To keep insects out of bags of grain and flour, add a couple of bay leaves to the containers.

‡ SWEET AND SALTY SUBSTITUTES

When substituting honey for sugar in a recipe, use a half cup of honey for every cup of sugar. Honey has about 65 calories per teaspoon; sugar has 45 calories per teaspoon. Since honey is twice as sweet as sugar, you need to use only half as much honey as sugar and so you save calories by using honey after all.

If salt is a no-no, use a spritz of lemon juice instead to help provide the kick that salt gives food.

‡ CLEANING STUFFED TOYS

Beanie Babies and other beloved stuffed toys are home to dust mites. Those dust mites can trigger allergic reactions such as asthma attacks. To kill those mighty mites, simply put the stuffed critter in a plastic bag and leave it in the freezer for twenty-four hours, once a week. Explain to your child that the stuffed toy joined the cast of *Holiday on Ice*, and it's "showtime" every Sunday or whenever.

‡ PRESCRIPTION READING MADE EASY

These are some of the Latin terms commonly used on prescriptions:

Term	Abbreviation	Meaning
ante cibum	ac	before food
bis in die	bid	twice a day
gutta	gt	drop
hora somni	hs	at bedtime
oculus dexter	od	right eye
oculus sinister	os	left eye
per os	po	by mouth
post cibum	pc	after food
pro re nata	prn	as needed
quaque 3 hora	q3h	every 3 hours
quaque die	qd	every day
quattuor in die	qid	4 times a day
ter in die	tid	3 times a day

‡ TAKING PILLS

Take pills standing up and keep standing for about two minutes afterward. Taking them with at least a half cup of water and while standing will give the pills a chance to move swiftly along, instead of staying in your esophagus where they may disintegrate and cause nausea or heartburn.

According to Dr. Stephen Paul of Temple University's School of Pharmacy, a multivitamin and fat-soluble vitamins A, D, and E should be taken with the largest meal of the day. That is when the greatest amount of fat is available in the stomach to aid the absorption of the vitamins.

The water-soluble vitamins—C and the B-complex—should be taken during a meal or a half hour before the meal. The vitamins help start the biochemical process that breaks down food, making it available to use for energy and tissue building.

If you take large doses of vitamin C, take it in small amounts throughout the day. Your body will use more of it that way, and you will help prevent urinary-tract irritation.

NOTE: NEVER take megadoses of any vitamins, minerals, or herbs unless you do so under the supervision of a health professional.

‡ DO-IT-YOURSELF ICE PACK AND HOT WATER BOTTLE

Don't throw away empty laundry room plastic containers. Next time you need a hot water bottle, fill one of those containers with hot water. Just be sure the cap is tight-fitting.

You know the plastic bottle with the tight-fitting cap that you used for a hot water bottle in the helpful hint above? Fill it with ice cold water and you have an ice pack.

You can make a flexible ice pack with a towel. Dunk a towel in cold water, wring it out, and place it on aluminum foil in the freezer. Before it freezes stiff, take it out of the freezer and mold it around the bruised or injured part of the body.

‡ STRENGTHEN YOUR IMMUNE SYSTEM

A daily serving of yogurt with "live cultures" seems to increase immune-enhancing chemicals, according to the results of experiments performed by George Halpern, M.D., of the department of internal medicine at the University of California, Davis, School of Medicine. Dr. Halpern emphasizes the need for the yogurt to contain "live" or "active cultures." Also check to see that the label says, "Contains L. acidophilus."

As an added bonus, the daily dose of yogurt may completely eliminate gas problems.

‡ BATHING MADE EASY

For those of you who can't stand long enough to take a shower, and who find it very hard to get up out of a bathtub once you've gotten into it, make the bathing/showering process easier by placing an aluminum beach chair in the tub. Turn on the shower and sit in the chair. Be sure to have those nonslip stick-ons on the floor of the tub.

‡ RAW GARLIC MADE EASY

The more we research and write about the benefits of garlic, the more garlic we want to eat. And we found a way to eat it so that we don't walk around with garlic breath. We mince the garlic cloves and drink them down in some water or orange juice. As long as we don't chew the little pieces of garlic, the smell doesn't linger.

You can also put a minced clove of garlic in applesauce, fat-free yogurt, or sour cream. It's delicious that way, and no one will know that you just ate raw garlic.

Incidentally, you may want to check out our book, *Garlic—Nature's Super Healer* (Prentice Hall).

A fast and easy way to peel a clove of garlic is to pound the clove with a blunt object—the side of a heavy knife, a rolling pin, or the bottom of a jar.

‡ GARLIC AND ONION ODORS ON HANDS

This helpful hint works like magic. Take a piece of silverware (any metal spoon, knife, or fork will do), pretend it's a cake of soap, and wash your hands with it under cold water. The garlic or onion smell will vanish in seconds.

Those pungent garlic and onion odors can also be removed by rubbing your hands with a slice of fresh tomato.

‡ GASOLINE ON HANDS

To get the smell of gasoline off your hands, rub them with salt.

‡ JAR SMELLS

In order to recycle jars, you may have to remove the odors left by its original contents. For a medium-size jar, use 1 teaspoon of dry mustard and fill it to the rim with water. Leave it that way for four to six hours, then rinse with hot water.

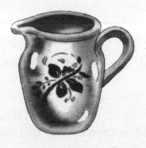

‡ WORKING WITH ONIONS, TEARLESSLY . . . ALMOST

In her search for a method of working with onions tearlessly, Joan has worn sunglasses, chewed white bread, let cold water run, frozen the onion first, and cut off the root end of the onion last.

Joan heard *Wheel of Fortune* letter-turner Vanna White thank the TV show's host, Pat Sajak, for this hint: Put a match, unlit, sulfur-side out, between your lips as though it were a cigarette. Keep it there while you peel, grate, or cut onions without worrying about your mascara running.

This hint is, by far, the best, but a really strong onion will still bring a tear to Joan's eye.

‡ HOLD ON TO YOUR PANTY HOSE

Onions and potatoes will keep better and longer if you store them in old nylon hose in a cool place. The hose allows the air to get to them.

‡ PESTICIDE REMOVAL FOR FRUITS AND VEGETABLES

Remove poisonous sprays and pesticides from produce using the Jay Kordich ("The Juiceman") method. Fill the sink with cold water and add 4 tablespoons of salt and the fresh juice of half a lemon. This makes a diluted form of hydrochloric acid. Soak most fruits and vegetables five to ten minutes; soak leafy greens two to three minutes; soak strawberries, blueberries, and all other berries one to two minutes. After soaking, rinse thoroughly in plain cold water, and enjoy.

Or you can soak produce in a sink or basin with ¼ cup of white vinegar. Then, with a vegetable brush, scrub the produce under cold water. Give them a final rinse, and they're ready to be eaten.

‡ NEED AN EYE-, EAR, OR NOSE DROPPER?

If you need a dropper *now* for any of your orifices, and don't have one, you may be able to improvise with a straw. A 3-inch piece of plastic straw will yield about 15 drops of liquid. Of course, that means you have to have a straw.

‡ FRESHEN UP A SICKROOM

Dip a puff of cotton into eucalyptus oil, put it on a little dish, and place it on a surface—not near an open window or a draft—in the room where someone is recovering. Eucalyptus oil is said to generate ozone. It's also a strong antiseptic. The oil has a powerful scent, so before you do this, be sure the person whose room you want to leave it in agrees to having it there.

‡ HERB AND SPICE STORAGE

Store herbs and spices in a cool, dry area. The refrigerator is ideal. When exposed to heat, like from the kitchen stove, spices and herbs lose their potency and their colors fade, too.

‡ NATURAL AIR POLLUTION CLEANERS

Your tax dollars have paid for National Aeronautics and Space Administration (NASA) research, and now you should and can benefit by it.

NASA's scientists discovered that several common houseplants can dramatically reduce toxic chemical levels in homes and offices. If you don't think your home or office is polluted, rethink it. There's benzene (found in inks, oils, paints, plastics, rubber, detergents, dyes, and gasoline); formaldehyde (found in foam insulation, particle board, pressed-wood products, most cleaning agents, and paper products treated with resins, including facial tissues and paper towels); and trichloroethylene (TCE, which is found in dry-cleaning processes, printing inks, paints, lacquers, varnishes, and adhesives).

Here are low-cost, attractive solutions in the form of hardy, easy-to-find, easy-to-grow household plants:

- Spider Plant *(Chlorophytum comosum "Vittatum")*—very easy to grow in indirect or bright-diffused light. Provide good drainage.
- Peace Lily *(Spathiphyllum species)*—very easy to grow in low-light location.
- Chinese Evergreen *(Aglaonema "Silver Queen")*—very easy to grow in low-light location. Remove overgrown shoots to encourage new growth, and keep the plant bushy.
- Weeping fig *(Ficus benjamina)*—easy to grow, but requires a little special attention. Indirect or bright-diffused light is best.
- Golden Pothos *(Epipremnum aureum)*—very easy to grow in indirect or bright-diffused light.

Moderately moist soil is preferred on all of these plants.

NASA recommends placing fifteen to eighteen plants in an 1,800-square-foot home. In a small to average-size room, one plant ought to do it, especially if it's placed where air circulates.

After the plants are in place, you, colleagues, and/or members of your household may find that sore throats, headaches, irritated eyes, and stuffy noses have cleared up.

The Ultimate Remedy

"Everyone needs at least three hugs a day in order to be healthy," claims Professor Sidney B. Simon of the University of Massachusetts.

According to Saint Ailred, "No medicine is more valuable, none more efficacious, none better suited to the cure of all our temporal ills than a friend."

Keeping those thoughts in mind, we figured out the Ultimate Remedy: Either hug three friends once a day, or hug one friend three times a day!

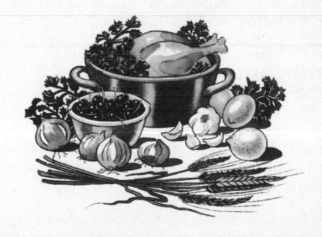

Recommended Reading

‡ **BRAIN POWER**
Brain Builders—A Lifelong Guide To Sharper Thinking, Better Memory and an Age-Proof Mind by Richard Leviton (Prentice Hall, 1995). Learn to maximize your brain's potential.

Ignite Your Intuition by Craig Korges (Health Communications, Inc., 1999). Learn to improve your memory, make better decisions, be more creative, and achieve your full potential.

Your Miracle Brain by Jean Carper (HarperCollins, 2000). New scientific evidence reveals how you can use food and supplements to maximize your brain power, boost your memory, lift your mood, improve IQ and creativity, and prevent and reverse mental aging.

‡ **FOLK AND HOME REMEDIES**
The Complete Self-Care Guide to Holistic Medicine—Treating Our Most Common Ailments by Robert S. Irker, D.O., Robert A. Anderson, M.D., and Larry Trivieri, Jr. (Jeremy P. Tarcher/Putnam, 1999). Alternative and conventional therapies that provide holistic treatment programs for more than sixty-five health challenges.

Doctor's Guide To Natural Medicine by Paul Barney, M.D. (Woodland Publishing, 1998). A complete and easy-to-use natural reference from a medical doctor's perspective. It includes alternative therapies, herbs, and supplements for over one hundred ailments.

Folk Remedies That Work by Joan Wilen & Lydia Wilen (HarperCollins, 1996). A useful, effective collection of safe, practical, doctor-approved new-age and age-old remedies.

Headaches by Robert Milne, M.D. and Blake More with Burton Goldberg (Future Medicine Publishing, Inc., 1997). Say goodbye to migraine, sinus, cluster, tension, food-related sensitivity, allergy, eyestrain, trauma, physical exertion, and rebound/stimulant-triggered headaches using natural alternative therapies.

More Chicken Soup & Other Folk Remedies by Joan Wilen & Lydia Wilen (Ballantine Books, 2000). This handy reference book will help you help yourself with life's everyday health challenges. Check out the Sensational 6 Superfoods—a new chapter that may change the way you eat, and how you feel.

Natural First Aid by Brigitte Mars, Herbalist AHG (Storey Books, 1999). Herbal treatments for ailments and injuries; emergency preparedness; and wilderness safety.

The Practical Encyclopedia of Sex and Health by Stefan Bechtel and the editors of *Men's Health* and *Prevention* magazines (Rodale, Inc., 1993). Over 120 fact-filled entries for enjoyment, safety, vitality, and love—from aphrodisiacs and hormones to potency, vasectomy, and yeast infection. (FYI: The book predates Viagra.)

Secrets of the Sacred White Buffalo by Gary Null, Ph.D. (Prentice Hall, 1998). Native American healing remedies, rites, and rituals to help you cleanse, heal, and live in harmony with the earth.

‡ FOODS, HEALTHFUL EATING, AND WEIGHT PROGRAMS

The Bone Density Diet—6 Weeks to a Strong Body and Mind by George J. Kessler, D.O., P.C., with Colleen Kapklein (Ballantine Books, 2000). This program reclaims bone density at any age; halts and reverses the aging process of the bones; boosts bone metabolism; and reduces stress and increases energy. Includes clear exercise illustrations along with food plan recipes.

Complete Candida Yeast Guidebook—Everything You Need to Know About Prevention, Treatment and Diet by Jeanne Marie Martin and Zoltan P. Roma, M.D. (Prima Publishing, 1996). Recipes included.

Eating Well For Optimum Health—The Essential Guide to Food, Diet and Nutrition by Andrew Weil, M.D. (Alfred A. Knopf, 2000). Basic information about making the right diet choices; specific diet advice; and eighty-five recipes.

The Enzyme Cure by Lita Lee, Ph.D., with Lisa Turner and Burton Goldberg (Future Medicine Publishing, Inc., 1998). A self-help program using plant enzymes to help you relieve or prevent any of thirty-six health problems.

Foods For Healing by Selene Yeager and the editors of *Prevention* health books (Rodale, Inc., 1998). Learn how one hundred common foods—from apricots and bananas, to wine and yogurt—can be used in sickness and in health.

Garlic—Nature's Super Healer by Joan Wilen & Lydia Wilen (Prentice Hall, 1997). Discover the amazing power of garlic through remedies, recipes, and lore.

Good Fat, Bad Fat by William P. Castelli, M.D., and Glen C. Griffin, M.D. (Fisher Books, 1997). A simple plan to reduce saturated fat, lower your cholesterol, and reduce your odds of a heart attack. Over 160 recipes included.

Is Your Thyroid Making You Fat? by Sanford Siegal, D.O., M.D. (Warner Books, Inc., 2000). Twenty-eight days to a life-changing diagnosis includes the doctor's breathrough home test.

Living Foods For Optimum Health by Brian R. Clement (Prima Publishing, 1998). Brian Clement, director of Hippocrates Health Institute in Florida, shares his years of experience teaching people to stay healthy in an unhealthy world.

10 Essential Foods by Lalitha Thomas (Hohm Press, 1997). In-depth nutritional information for vitality, health, and well-being, plus tips and some recipes.

3 Days to Vitality by Pamela Serure (HarperCollins, 1998). Cleanse your body; clear your mind; claim your spirit—all that in just three days.

Vegetarian's A–Z Guide to Fruits and Vegetables by Kathleen Robinson, with Pete Luckett (Fisher Books, 1996). This enlightening guide is not only for vegetarians, but for anyone who wants to add more fruits and vegetables to their diet.

Weight Loss by Burton Goldberg and the editors of *Alternative Medicine* (Alternative Medicine Company, 2000). This is not just another diet book. It has seventeen smart ways to permanently shed unwanted pounds, with input from twenty-five doctors.

‡ HERBS

Dr. Duke's Essential Herbs by James A. Duke, Ph.D. (Rodale, Inc., 1999). From one of the world's most respected botanists, here are thirteen vital herbs you need to disease-proof your body, boost your energy, and lengthen your life.

Herbal Healing Secrets of the Orient by Darlena L'Orange, I.Ac. (Prentice Hall, 1998). Learn to use the healing power of the 108 Oriental herbs that are the foundation of Chinese medicine.

The Herbal Home Remedy Book by Joyce A. Wardwell (Storey Books, 1998). Simple recipes for tinctures, teas, salves, tonics, and syrups, and inspiration to make you want to grow your own herbs.

‡ JUST FOR MEN
Body Care Just For Men by Jun Long (Storey Books, 1999). Natural health tips and herbal formulas for skin protection, sore muscle relief, aftershaves, tonics, and more.

‡ JUST FOR WOMEN
The Living Beauty Detox Program—The Revolutionary Diet for Each and Every Season of A Woman's Life by Ann Louise Gittleman, M.S., C.N.S. (HarperCollins, 2000). This gifted nutritionist tells how to cleanse yourself of toxins, manage your hormones, and look your best.

‡ NEW-AGE AND AGE-OLD (MOSTLY ALTERNATIVE) THERAPIES
Alternative Medicine: The Definitive Guide compiled by The Burton Goldberg Group (Future Medicine Publishing, 1994). This huge book is brimming with over four hundred leading alternative health professionals who share their effective therapies.

Aromatherapy—A Lifetime Guide To Healing With Essential Oils by Valerie Gennarie Cooksley (Prentice Hall, 1996). A step-by-step, hands-on guide to good health using the curative power of essential oils.

Creative Visualization—Using Imagery and Imagination for Self Transformation by Ronald Shone (Destiny Books, 1998). Improve your health, raise your energy level, and relieve pain—all using deep relaxation and visualization.

The Essential Flower Essence Handbook by Lila Devi (Hay House, Inc., 1996). Remedies for inner well-being with vibrational flower therapy by a respected flower essence researcher, practitioner, and teacher.

Growing Older, Growing Better by Amy E. Dean (Hay House, Inc., 1997). Daily meditations, affirmations, commonsense suggestions, and lots of reasons for celebrating age.

Magnet Therapy—The Pain Cure Alternative by Ron Lawrence, M.D., Ph.D., Paul J. Rosch, M.D., F.A.C.P., and Judith Plowden (Prima Publishing, 1998). Learn about the therapeutic benefits of magnets from outstanding experts in the field.

Nature's Cures by Michael Castleman (Rodale, Inc., 1996). From acupressure and aromatherapy, to walking and yoga, this guide has scientifically proven, drug-free healing methods.

Prayer, Faith and Healing—Cure Your Body, Heal Your Mind and Restore Your Soul by Kenneth Winston Caine and Brian Paul Kaufman (Rodale Press, 1999). Over five hundred ways to use the power of belief, from America's leading pastors, counselors, doctors, and health researchers.

Sounds of Healing by Mitchell L. Gaynor, M.D. (Broadway Books, 1999). Dr. Gaynor is an oncologist and director of integrative medicine at the Strang-Cornell Cancer Prevention Center. He has been using *sound* as complementary therapy with remarkable results. This book has self-healing techniques for everything from minor daily stresses to life-threatening challenges.

Urine Therapy by Flora Peschek-Bohmar, Ph.D., and Gisela Schreiber (Healing Arts Press, 1999). Using your own urine to treat common ailments including acne, asthma, hair loss, indigestion, migraines, warts, wrinkles, and more.

Your Body Can Talk by Susan L. Levy, D.C., and Carol Lehr, M.A. (Hohm Press, 1996). Using simple muscle testing, you can learn what your body knows and needs for health and well-being.

‡ PETS
New Choices in Natural Healing For Dogs & Cats by Amy D. Shojai and the editors of *Prevention for Pets* (Rodale, Inc., 1999). Over one thousand at-home remedies for your pet's problems using herbs, acupressure, massage, homeopathy, flower essences, natural diets, and healing energy.

‡ SPECIFIC HEALTH CHALLENGES
Definitive Guide to Cancer by W. John Diamond, M.D., and W. Lee Cowdown, M.D., with Burton Goldberg (Future Medicine Publishing, Inc., 1997). Cancer can be reversed. This important, lifesaving book tells how, using clinically proven complementary and alternative therapies. Thirty-seven physicians explain their proven, safe, nontoxic, and successful treatments for reversing cancer.

Live Now, Age Later by Isadore Rosenfeld, M.D. (Warner Books, 1999). Proven ways to slow down the clock by preventing or treating specific conditions like Alzheimer's, cancer, constipation, heart disease, impotence, osteoporosis, and more.

7 Weeks To Emotional Healing by Joan Mathews Larson, Ph.D. (Ballantine Books, 1999). Proven natural formulas for eliminating depression, anxiety, fatigue, and anger from your life.

‡ VITAMINS AND OTHER SUPPLEMENTS

The Supplement Shopper by Gregory Pouls, D.C., and Maile Pouls, Ph.D., with Burton Goldberg (Future Medicine Publishing, Inc., 1999). This guide may help you take the guesswork out of choosing the best supplement for whatever ails you. It has the kind of information you should be discussing with your doctor.

Vitamins, Herbs, Minerals & Supplements by H. Winter Griffith, M.D. (Fisher Books, 1998). User-friendly format that can give you answers about supplements and help you use them most efficiently.

Sources

‡ HERBAL PRODUCTS AND MORE

Atlantic Spice Company
2 Shore Road
P.O. Box 205
North Truro, MA 02652
Note: Wholesale to the public.

Free Catalog
Tel: 800 / 316-7965
Fax: 508 / 487-2550
Website: www.atlantic
spice.com

Blessed Herbs
109 Barre Plains Road
Oakham, MA 01068

Free Catalog
Tel: 800 / 489-4372
Fax: 508 / 882-3755
Email: blessedherbs@
blessedherbs.com

Dial Herbs
P.O. Box 39
Fairview, UT 84629

Free Catalog
Tel: 800 / 288-4618
    435 / 427-9476
Fax: 435 / 427-9448
Website: www.dialdist.com

Flower Power Herbs and
    Roots Inc.
406 East 9th Street
New York, NY 10009

Tel: 212 / 982-6664
Website: www.flowerpower.net

Great American Natural
    Products
4121 16th Street North
St. Petersburg, FL 33703

Free Catalog
Tel: 800 / 323-4372
Fax: 727 / 522-6457

Haussmann's Herbs &
  Naturals
220 Market Street
Philadelphia, PA 19102

Free Catalog
Tel: 800 / 235-5522
    215 / 627-1168
Fax: 215 / 629-0339

Indiana Botanic Gardens
P.O. Box 5
Hammond, IN 46325

Free Catalog
Tel: 800 / 644-8327
    219 / 947-4040
Fax: 219 / 947-4148
Website: www.botanic
  health.com

Mountain Top Herbs, Inc.
P.O. Box 970004
Orem, UT 84097 0004

Tel: 877 / KIT-TALK
        (548-8255)
Website: www.herbkit.com

Nature's Apothecary
1558 Cherry Street
Louisville, CO 80027

Free Catalog
Tel: 800 / 999-7422
    303 / 664-1600
Fax: 303 / 664-5106
Website: www.natures
  apothecary.com

New Chapter, Inc.
P.O. Box 1947
22 High Street
Brattleboro, VT 05301

Free Catalog
Tel: 800 / 543-7279
    802 / 257-0018
Fax: 802 / 257-0018
Website: www.new-chapter.com

Old Amish Herbal Remedies
4141 Irish Street North
St. Petersburg, FL 33703

Free Catalog
Tel: 813 / 521-4372
Fax: 727 / 522-6457

Penn Herb Co. Ltd.
10601 Decatur Road
Philadelphia, PA 19123

Free Catalog
Tel: 800 / 523-9971
Fax: 215 / 632-7945
Website: www.pennherb.com

San Francisco Herb Company
250 14th Street
San Francisco, CA 94103
Note: Wholesale to the
    public.

Free Catalog
Tel: 800 / 227-4530
Fax: 415 / 861-4440
Website: www.sfherb.com

‡ GEMS AND NEW AGE PRODUCTS AND GIFTS

Beyond the Rainbow
P.O. Box 110
Ruby, NY 12475

Tel: 914 / 336-4609
Fax: 914 / 336-0953
Website:
    www.rainbowcrystal.com

Crystal Way
2335 Market Street
San Francisco, CA 94114

Tel: 800 / 453-HEAL (4325)
    415 / 861-6511
Fax: 415 / 861-4229
Website: www.crystalway.com

Divine Intervention
5800 Main Street #270
Hesperia, CA 92345

Tel: 800 / 863-3442
Fax: 760 / 947-4093
Website: www.divine
    intervention.com

Pacific Spirit
1334 Pacific Avenue
Forest Grove, OR 97116

Free Catalog
Tel: 800 / 634-9057
Fax: 503 / 357-1669
Website: www.
    mystictrader.com

‡ VITAMINS, NUTRITIONAL SUPPLEMENTS, AND MORE

Freeda Vitamins
36 East 41st Street
New York, NY 10017
Note: All products are

Free Catalog
Tel: 800 / 777-3737
    212 / 685-4980
Fax: 212 / 685-7297

100 percent kosher, yeast-free, vegetarian- and Feingold-approved for hyperactive children.

Website: www.freeda
vitamins.com

L&H Vitamins
32–33 47th Avenue
Long Island City, NY 11101

Free Catalog
Tel: 800 / 221-1152
Fax: 718 / 472-5499
Website: www.vitamins.com

Nature's Distributors, Inc.
16508 E. Laser Drive,
Building B
Fountain Hills, AZ
85268-6512

Free Catalog
Tel: 800 / 624-7114
Fax: 480 / 837-8420
Website: www.natures
distributors.com

NutriCology Inc.
30806 Santana Street
Hayward, CA 94544

Free Catalog
Tel: 800 / 545-9960
Fax: 510 / 487-8682
Website: www.nutricology.com

Nutrition Coalition, Inc.
P.O. Box 3001
Fargo, ND 58108

Free Information on
Willard Water
Tel: 800 / 447-4793
Fax: 218 / 236-6753
Website: www.willards
water.com

Puritan's Pride
1233 Montauk Highway
P.O. Box 9001
Oakdale, NY 11769-9001

Free Catalog
Tel: 800 / 645-1030
Fax: 631 / 471-5693
Website: www.puritan.com

Superior Nutritionals Inc.
1150 94th Avenue North
St. Petersburg, FL 33702
Specializes in well-researched, high-quality, physician-tested products.

Tel: 800 / 717-RUNN (7866)
727 / 577-4344
Fax: 727 / 577-3166

TriMedica, International
1895 So. Los Feliz Drive
Tempe, AZ 85281

Free Catalog
Tel: 800 / 800-8849
Fax: 480 / 346-3191
Website: www.trimedica.com

The Vitamin Shoppe
4700 Westside Avenue
North Bergen, NJ 07047

Free Catalog
Tel: 800 / 223-1216
Fax: 800 / 852-7153
Website: www.vitamin
shoppe.com

‡ NATURAL FOODS AND MORE

Barlean's Organic Oils
4936 Lake Terrell Road
Ferndale, WA 98248

Free Catalog &
Flax Oil Information
Tel: 800 / 445-FLAX (3529)
Fax: 800 / 551-9879
Website: www.barleans.com

Crusoe Island Natural Foods
267 Rt. 89 South
Savannah, NY 13146-9711

Free Catalog
Tel: 800 / 724-2233
315 / 365-3949
Fax: 315 / 365-2690
Website: www.crusoeisland.com

Gold Mine Natural Food Co.
7805 Arjons Drive
San Diego, CA 92126

Free Catalog
Tel: 800 / 475-FOOD (3663)
Fax: 858 / 695-0811
Website: www.goldmine
naturalfood.com

Jaffe Bros. Natural
Foods, Inc.
P.O. Box 636, Dept. JL
Valley Center, CA
92082-0636

Free Catalog
Tel: 760 / 749-1133
Fax: 760 / 749-1282
Website: www.organic
fruitsandnuts.com

‡ BEE PRODUCTS AND MORE

C.C. Pollen
3627 E. Indian School Road–
  Suite 209
Phoenix, AZ 85018-5126

Free Literature & Product List
Tel: 800 / 875-0096
  602 / 957-0096
Fax: 602 / 381-3130
Website: www.ccpollen.com

Health from the Hive
Bee Supplies & Products
James Hagemeyer, Beekeeper
  (known as "Mr. Bee Pollen")
5337 Highway 411
Madisonville, TN 37354

Tel: 423 / 442-2038
Website: www.healthfrom
  thehive.com

Montana Naturals
19994 Highway 93
Arlee, MT 59821

Tel: 800 / 872-7218
Fax: 800 / 239-4819

‡ PET FOOD AND PRODUCTS

Golden Tails
6509 Transit Road, Suite 82
Bowmansville, NY 14026

Tel: 716 / 681-6986
Fax: 716 / 681-6958
Website: www.goldentails.com

Halo Purely for Pets
3438 East Lake Road, #14
Palm Harbor, FL 34685

Free Catalog & Animal Care
  Booklet
Tel: 800 / 426-4256
Fax: 813 / 891-6328
Website: www.halopets.com

Harbingers of a New Age
717 East Missoula Avenue
Troy, MT 59935-9609

Free Catalog
Tel: 800 / 884-6262
Fax: 406 / 295-7603
Website: www.montana
  sky.net/vegepet

The Natural Pet Care Co.
8050 Lake City Way
Seattle, WA 98115

Free Catalog
Tel: 800 / 962-8266
206 / 522-1667
Fax: 206 / 522-1132
Website: www.allthe
    bestpetcare.com

‡ HEALTH-RELATED PRODUCTS

Inner Balance—Natural
    Solutions For Health
360 Interlocken Blvd.,
Suite 300
Broomfield, CO 80021

Free Catalog
Tel: 800 / 482-3608
Fax: 800 / 456-1139
Website: www.gaiam.com

InteliHealth Healthy Home
97 Commerce Way
P.O. Box 7007
Dover, DE 19903

Free Catalog
Tel: 800 / 988-1127
Fax: 800 / 676-3299
Website: www.intelihealth.com

Perfect Balance for Mind,
    Body and Soul
7101 Winnetka Avenue N
P.O. Box 9437
Minneapolis, MN 55440-9437

Free Catalog
Tel: 800 / 729-9000
Website: www.damark.com

Self Care Catalog
104 Challenger Drive
Portland, TN 37148

Free Catalog
Tel: 800 / 345-3371
Fax: 800 / 345-4021
Website: www.selfcare.com

‡ HEALTH-RELATED TRAVEL PRODUCTS AND MORE

Magellan's
(Essentials for the Traveler)

Free Catalog
Tel: 800 / 962-4943

110 West Sola Street
Santa Barbara, CA 93101

Fax: 805 / 568-5406
Website: www.
    magellans.com

‡ MACROBIOTIC FOODS AND SPECIALTY COOKWARE

Macrobiotic Company of
    America
799 Old Leicester Highway
Asheville, NC 28806

Free Catalog
Tel: 800 / 438-4730
Fax: 828 / 252-9479
Website: www.mountain
    ark.com

‡ WHOLESALE/RETAIL HEALTH APPLIANCES

Acme Equipment
1024 Concert Avenue
Spring Hill, FL 34609

Free Catalog
Tel: 800 / 201-0706
Fax: 352 / 683-7740

‡ AROMATHERAPY, FLOWER ESSENCES, AND MORE

Aromaland
1326 Rufina Circle
Santa Fe, NM 87505

Free Catalog
Tel: 800 / 933-5267
Fax: 505 / 438-7223
Website: www.aromaland.com

Aroma Vera
5901 Rodeo Road
Los Angeles, CA 90016

Free Catalog
Tel: 800 / 669-9514
    310 / 280-0407
Fax: 310 / 204-2746
Website: www.aromavera.com

Flower Essence Services
P.O. Box 1769

Free Catalog
Tel: 800 / 548-0075

Nevada City, CA 05050

530 / 265-0258
Fax: 530 / 265-6467
Website: www.flower
essence.com

‡ SERVICES

Ailment Information Including Holistic Alternatives
La Verne and Steve Ross are cofounders of the World Research Foundation. They have an incredible service. For a
nominal fee, they will do a search (which includes five thousand international medical journals) and provide you with
the newest holistic and conventional treatments and diag-
nostic techniques on most any condition. The foundation's
library of more than ten thousand books, periodicals, and
research reports is available to the public free of charge.
Write, call, fax, or visit their Website.

World Research Foundation   Tel: 520 / 284-3300
41 Bell Rock Plaza   Fax: 520 / 284-3530
Sedona, AZ 86351   Website: www.wrf.org

Product Safety
The U.S. Consumer Product Safety Commission has an
around-the-clock hot line with information on harmful products. With paper and pen in hand, call: 800 / 638-2772;
Maryland residents call: 800 / 492-8104.

Check Up on Specialists
The American Board of Medical Specialties has a toll-free
number for you to call when you want to make sure that
a "specialist" is just that. When you call, give them the
doctor's name, and they will tell you whether the doctor
is listed in a specialty and the year of certification. Call
weekdays, between 9 A.M. and 6 P.M. EST: 800 / 776-CERT
(2378).

Take Advantage of Your Tax Dollars

The Consumer Information Catalog lists more than two hundred free and low-cost publications from Uncle Sam—on everything from saving money, staying healthy and getting federal benefits, to buying a home and handling consumer complaints.

There are three easy ways to get your free copy of the catalog:

- Call toll-free: 888 / 8-PUEBLO (878-3256), weekdays 9 A.M. to 8 P.M. EST.
- Send your name and address to Consumer Information Catalog, Pueblo, CO 81009.
- Go on-line to check out and order the catalog through the Consumer Information Center's Website at www.pueblo.gsa.gov. While you're there, you can read, print out, or download any CIC publication for free.

‡ HEALTH-RELATED WEBSITES

Before we start www-ing down the page, there's something you should know, and probably already do: You can't always trust the information you get on the Internet. Since we're talking about "your health," it can be mighty dangerous to accept and use wrong advice. Our advice is to take whatever information you get on-line that seems appropriate for your condition, and show it to and/or discuss it with your health professional.

There's something else you may already know, but if not, you should. There's an organization called the HON (Health On the Net) Foundation (www.hon.ch), associated with the University Hospitals of Geneva. HON is like the Better Business Bureau for medical Websites. Their prestigious governing body certifies sites that abide by eight user-protecting principles. So, if HON gives a site its stamp of approval, you will see it on the site, and while you may be able to trust the integrity of the information a bit more, still be sure to check out any and all advice with your health professional.

HON is not the only organization certifying Websites. There's the Internet Healthcare Coalition (www.ihc.net) and Health Internet Ethics (Hi-Ethics), founded in part by former surgeon general C. Everett Koop (www.health wise.org/Hi-EthicsHome.htm).

At these three Websites, you'll find direct links to established (and certified, of course) health sites—many of the ones listed below.

www.americanheart.org
American Heart Association National Center
Education and information on fighting heart disease and stroke

www.arfa.org
The American Running Association
News, tips, articles, membership information, fitness links, and free sample Running and FitNews newsletter

www.askdrweil.com (or) www.drweil.com
Dr. Andrew Weil answers health questions asked by emailers
User-friendly archives

www.cancer.org
American Cancer Society
Education and information

www.certifieddoctor.org
On-line version of American Board of Medical Specialists Public Education Program's physician locator and information service

www.chid.nih.gov/
Combined Health Information Database, National Institutes of Health, Centers For Disease Control and Prevention, Health Resources and Services Administration

www.clinicaltrials.gov
A service of the National Institutes of Health
Current information about clinical research studies
Links patients to medical research

www.eFit.com
Health and fitness site with lots going on
Free personalized weight management, nutrition and exercise program
Type in your zip code and find the closest gyms and healthy-menu restaurants.

www.familydoctor.co.nz
Health information by practicing doctors

www.fda.gov
Food and Drug Administration

www.healthfinder.gov
Department of Health and Human Services
The site is linked to other agencies and self-help and support groups

www.healthweb.org
Provides links to specific evaluated information resources selected by librarians and professionals at leading academic medical centers in the Midwest

www.healthyideas.com
Prevention's Website has herbal remedies, vitamin databases, alternative medicine news, advice from naturopathic doctors, and lots more.

www.kidshealth.org
Created by pediatric medical experts at the Alfred I. duPont Hospital for Children, and other children's nationwide health facilities

www.mealsforyou.com
Thousands of recipes, meal plans, and complete nutritional information. Look up recipes by name, ingredient, or nutrition—recipes adjust for number of servings.

www.merck.com
Searchable on-line version of the Merck Manual of Medical Information

www.nlm.nib.gov/medlineplus
National Library of Medicine's Medline Plus
Health information selected by the National Library of Medicine from a database of more than four thousand medical journals

www.oncolink.upenn.edu
The University of Pennsylvania's cancer information site with related information links

www.siu.edu/departments/bushea
Your Health Is Your Business
Links to many healthsites

www.soyfoods.com
Monthly newsletter, soy research information, U.S. soyfoods directory, recipe books, food manufacturing information

www.talksoy.com
Soy recipes and health and nutrition information

www.wellweb.com
Wellness web
A comprehensive health and medical information clearing-house, including conventional and alternative medicine, nutrition, fitness, and late-breaking medical research.

www.wunderlichcenter.com
Dr. Ray C. Wunderlich, Jr., known as "The Real Doctor" in honor of his pioneering contributions in the alternative medicine movement, is dedicated to promoting nutritional and preventive medicine at the Wunderlich Center for Nutritional Medicine in St. Petersburg, Florida. The Website has his informative and humorous health articles.

Index